Baby & Me

Guide to Pregnancy and Newborn Care

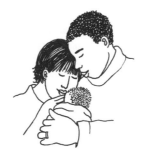

Fourth edition, 2006

Written by Deborah D. Stewart

Illustrated by Christine Thomas

Published by Bull Publishing Company

Bull Publishing Company
P.O. Box 1377
Boulder, CO 80306
Phone: 800-676-2855
www.bullpub.com

The material in this publication is for general information only and is not intended to provide specific advice or medical recommendations for any individual. Your doctor or other health professional must be consulted for the advice with regard to your individual situation.

Library of Congress Cataloging-in-Publication Data

Stewart, Deborah D.
  Baby & me : guide to pregnancy and newborn care / written by
Deborah D. Stewart ; illustrated by Christine Thomas. — 4th ed.
      p. cm.
  Includes index.
  ISBN-13: 978-0-923521-90-5
  ISBN-10: 0-923521-90-9
1. Pregnancy—Popular works. 2. Childbirth—Popular works.
I. Title. II. Title: Baby and me.

  RG525.S693 2006
  618.2—dc22

                                                   2006015439

To my grandson,
Stewart James McCleary,
Who just turned three and lights up my life,
every day

I want to thank all those who helped me make this edition the best it can be, especially Mike Gold, who was my constant support person through a very prolonged labor and delivery.

Reviewers of the new edition who made many helpful suggestions: Linda S. Ungerleider, RN, MSN, coauthor of my infant care book, *Best Start*; Ellen Mann, CNM, Portland, OR; Mark Hathaway, MD, Washington Hospital Center, Washington, DC; Jeanette Zaichkin, RNC, MN, Olympia, WA; and Barbara Leese, Portland, OR, new mother of two.

Many thanks to childbirth educators in Seattle who opened their classes to me: Carol Kauppila and Christine Wallace, Northwest Hospital; and Penny Swanson, Childbirth Education, Swedish Medical Ctr./Ballard.

I also appreciated and took to heart the useful comments on the previous edition made by Chris Ann Carion, RN, MSN, Gateway Health Plan, Pittsburgh, PA; Nancy Hunger, MVP Health Care, Schenectady, NY; Laura Richter, Womens' Gynecology and Childbirth Associates, Rochester, NY; and Deborah Oldakowski, MCH Education Coordinator, St. Luke's Hospital, Cedar Rapids, IA.

A message to you from me...

I know how much parents' health habits can affect a child. My baby—now a strong young woman—was a tiny premature infant 36 years ago. My husband, our families, and I all worried through her long stay in the hospital. We feared that she might have lasting health problems. If I had known many of the things I know now, she might not have been born so early.

I wrote this book to help you stay healthy during pregnancy and keep your newborn healthy. The more you can do to prevent health problems the better, for yourself and your baby. The book will give you the basic information about pregnancy, birth, and caring for your new baby. It also will help you find more information when you need it.

I hope you will enjoy this special time in your life. Your body is doing an amazing job. It has the power to grow and protect new life. Keep this book to remember this time after your baby grows up. You will find places to make notes of special things you experience during pregnancy and after your baby's birth.

Good health is one of the best gifts a parent can give a child. *Baby & Me* should encourage you to do all you can for your child. Caring for yourself and your baby is a big task. You deserve plenty of help to make it easier.

Best wishes to you and your baby!

Deborah Davis Stewart

Seattle, Washington

April 2006

Table of Contents

Chapters and Topics	Page
1. Get Ready for Pregnancy	**1**
Health before pregnancy	2
Signs of pregnancy	6
2. Now You're Pregnant—What's Next?	**9**
First weeks of pregnancy	10
Important first steps	12
Father or partner's role	14
3. Staying Healthy	**17**
Daily living	22
Home and workplace	26
Mental health	28
4. What You Eat, Drink, and Breathe	**31**
Healthy eating	32
Things that can harm your baby	38
5. Medical Care During Pregnancy and Childbirth	**47**
Where will your baby be born?	48
Prenatal checkups	51
A doctor for your baby	53
6. Birth and Newborn Care—What You Need to Know Now	**55**
Learn about childbirth choices	56
Infant care, feeding, and equipment	61
7. First Trimester: Months 1, 2, and 3	**71**
Months 1 and 2	73
Month 3	82
8. Second Trimester: Months 4, 5, and 6	**91**
Month 4	92
Month 5	98
Month 6	103
9. Third Trimester: Months 7, 8, and 9	**107**
Month 7	109
Month 8	112

Month 9   122

10. **Your Baby's Birth**   **127**
Be prepared   128
Labor   136
Delivery   143

11. **Basic Newborn Care—Holding, Bathing, and More**   **149**
First day basics   151
Baby with special needs   161

12. **Feeding Your Newborn**   **163**
Basics   164
Breastfeeding   166
Bottlefeeding   174

13. **Getting to Know Your Baby**   **177**
Understanding your baby   180
How your baby develops   182
Sleep and crying   186

14. **Keeping Your Baby Safe**   **189**
Sleep safety and SIDS   190
Car seat safety   193
Falls, burns, baby-proofing   196

15. **Keeping Your Baby Healthy**   **199**
Keeping your baby healthy   199
Immunizations   202
Signs of illness   207

16. **Taking Care of Yourself**   **213**
As your body heals   214
Your 6-week checkup   218
Family planning   219
Depression after childbirth   220

17. **Resources to Help You**   **223**
Organizations   224
Books   228
Glossary of words   229

Index   **237**

Using this book

If you are already pregnant or planning to have a baby soon...

Taking care of yourself now is the most important thing you can do to have a healthy, happy baby. This book can help you do this. Now is a good time to take a quick look all the way through it. Keep it where you can find it easily. I hope you will use it often.

Fathers and others

This book is also for and about fathers and partners, and even grandparents. It can help them understand what is happening to you. I hope you will share it with them.

A book to write in

This is a book you can write in as much as you like! Keep notes about how you feel and questions you want to remember to ask at your next checkup. Write down special things you want to remember, like when you first feel your baby kick or hear the heart beat, in the record pages. You will enjoy looking back at these pages and remembering this special time. Record pages are in Chapters 9 and 10 and at the end of the book.

Family or traditional health habits

Health advice in this book may be different from what your family or your people have done in the past. For example, in some cultures, certain foods are not eaten during pregnancy. In others, the baby's father usually does not take part in the birth.

There are many ways to good health. The ideas in this book will give you and your baby a good chance for a healthy start. **If you want to do**

things differently, talk about it with your doctor, nurse, or nurse-midwife.

Special words

Because some babies are girls and some are boys, I take turns using "he" and "she" to mean any baby. In the same way, I may use "she" or "he" to refer to a doctor, nurse, or nurse-midwife.

You may hear the words "health care provider" or "provider" used in the clinic or by your health plan to refer to doctors or nurse-midwifes. I have used those words in some places, too.

I have tried to use as few medical words as possible. You may need to learn the ones you read here, because your doctor or nurse-midwife will probably use them. You will find their meanings on the page where they first appear or in the glossary at the back of the book. When you see a word marked like this (*), its meaning is at the side of the page.

Please note: This book should not be the only guide you use to care for yourself and your unborn child. Your doctor or nurse-midwife and other medical professionals are trained to help you take care of yourself. Please consult those who know your special needs.

Chapter 1

Get Ready for Pregnancy

Preparing yourself for a baby

Are you having sex?

Are you thinking about having a baby?

Do you think you might be pregnant?

It is never too soon to make your body a healthy home for an unborn baby.

Before you get pregnant is the best time to make sure your body is ready. But women often get pregnant when they are not expecting it. If you are already pregnant, start taking care of yourself right away. This way, your unborn baby will have a safe place to grow.

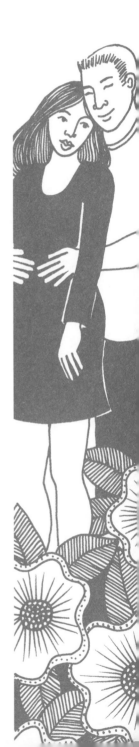

This chapter includes:

Health before pregnancy, page 2

- Your health history
- Healthy habits

Signs of pregnancy, page 6

- How to get a pregnancy test

Every woman wants to have a healthy baby. Most babies are born healthy, but some have health problems. Some problems can be prevented by what you do now. Many others can be made less serious.

Nobody likes to think about problems. However, nobody wants to learn too late that there was something they could have done to prevent a problem. Preventing a problem is better and easier than trying to fix it later.

Start out right before pregnancy

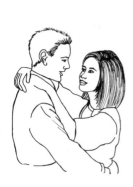

If possible, plan to get pregnant when you are ready to care for a baby. You and your child both will have a better life if you are healthy. It also is very important to have loving support from a partner, family, and friends.

Some problems begin in the first days after pregnancy begins, before a woman knows she is pregnant. Others happen as the baby grows. Pregnancy also can affect a woman's health condition, such as diabetes or high blood pressure.

Whatever your situation, you can make your body ready to be a healthy home for an unborn child.

How healthy are you now?

Your habits, your health, and your family's health history can affect your baby. The items below could give you problems during pregnancy or cause your baby to be born too early. Knowing about them now means you can do everything possible to keep yourself and your baby healthy.

Check any items below that are true for you.

Lifestyle:

____ I rarely eat fruits or vegetables three times a day.

____ I diet often or think I am too fat or too thin.

____ I smoke cigarettes.

____ I drink more than one glass of beer, wine, wine cooler, or hard liquor every week.

____ I am younger than 18 or older than 34.

____ I take medicines often.

____ I have used illegal drugs.

____ I work with x-rays, dangerous chemicals, or lead.

Health History:

____ I have diabetes, seizures, or high blood pressure.

____ I have or have had a sexually transmitted disease (STD), like herpes, chlamydia, gonorrhea, syphilis, or HIV/AIDS.

____ I have had problems during a pregnancy or have had a baby who weighed less than 5 1/2 pounds at birth.

____ I have had a miscarriage (lost a pregnancy).

____ Someone in my family has had a serious birth defect or problems during pregnancy.

____ Someone in my family has an illness that is passed from parent to child, like cystic fibrosis, hemophilia, sickle cell disease, or Tay-Sachs disease.

Tell your health care provider about all items you have checked. Learn how they could affect your baby. You could do something to stop or correct most of them. **What you do can make a big difference to your baby!**

Healthy habits before pregnancy

Many pregnancies are a surprise. If you are having sex, you could get pregnant. You will not know you are pregnant right away.

Important parts of your baby's body start to grow in the first days after conception. Anything that harms the tiny embryo in your uterus at this time can do serious damage before you know you are pregnant. That is why it is so important to make your body healthy before you get pregnant.

"It's amazing.... I had no idea how fast a baby starts developing. Nobody told me how careful I should be before I got pregnant."

Steps to take now:

- **Take a vitamin pill with folic acid every day.** Every woman needs to get enough folic acid every day to prevent birth defects. (See page 5.)

- **Ask your doctor about the effects any prescription drugs you take** could have on pregnancy.

- **Stop using alcohol, tobacco, and any illegal drugs.** Any time you smoke, drink alcohol, or use street drugs, your baby gets a dose, too. If you have trouble stopping, ask for help. You can quit!

- **Eat healthy foods.** Your body needs plenty of milk, fruits, vegetables, whole grains, and water. This is a good time to learn healthy eating habits. (See Chapter 4.)

- **Get any health problems under control.** Conditions like diabetes and high blood pressure could affect your pregnancy. Get health care now.

- **Get your body weight to a healthy level.** If you are too thin, your baby could be born early. If you are too heavy, your baby's health and your own could be in danger. A dietician could help you.

- **Talk with your partner** about your feelings about having a baby. Make sure you have his support before you get pregnant.

- **Learn about pregnancy.** Read this book and others. Ask questions about things you do not understand.

See Chapters 2, 3, and 4 for more details about living a healthy life.

Share these steps with your partner or husband. Also tell your girl friends, so they will be healthy before they get pregnant. Also make sure they know about and use birth control if they are not ready to have a baby.

Protecting your baby's fragile body

The brain and spinal cord* are the most important parts of every person's nervous system. They control how you think and move. The spinal cord and brain begin to grow in the first few weeks of life. It is easy to damage them without intending to.

You can help prevent brain and spinal cord problems. Do these things before you get pregnant or as soon as you think you might be pregnant.

Spinal cord:
The main nerve that carries messages about feeling and movement between your brain and body. It goes down your back inside the spine.

Avoid alcohol, cigarettes, and other drugs

Beer, wine, and hard liquor affect the growth of a baby's brain. The effect of alcohol on an unborn baby's brain is the main cause of mental retardation. Even one drink might cause harm—no one knows how much is safe. You can prevent this damage by not drinking.

Cigarette use slows an unborn baby's growth. It can lead to preterm (premature) birth*. Other drugs also can cause addiction, preterm birth, or mental problems. Protecting your baby is a great reason to quit! (See pages 42 through 46.)

Preterm birth:
Early birth, before 37 weeks. The premature infant usually is small and may need to stay in the hospital after birth. Many babies born very early have other health problems.

Get enough folic acid every day

Folic acid is a B vitamin that is important for everyone's health. It helps prevent very serious brain and spinal defects in babies. Talk with your doctor if you are not sure you should take folic acid.

Some of these defects happen in the very early days of pregnancy, before women know they are pregnant. Every teenage girl and woman who could get pregnant should get at least 0.4 milligrams (400 mcg) of folic acid every day.

Taking a multi-vitamin pill with folic acid every day is the easiest, best way to get enough folic acid. You can get some of this vitamin from foods, but you would need to eat very large amounts to get enough. Some foods that have a lot of folic acid are dark leafy green vegetables, broccoli, orange juice, bread, pasta, cereals, kidney beans and liver. Check the label on vitamin pills for folate, which is the same as folic acid.

If you do not like taking vitamin pills or if they are expensive, think about how important it is for any baby to have a healthy brain. And ask yourself if you always eat right. One option is to take folic acid pills. They are smaller and less expensive than multi-vitamin pills.

Tell your girlfriends about how important folic acid is for their future children. Let them know that they need to take it before they get pregnant.

*Spina bifida:
A very serious defect of the spine. It often prevents a person from walking.

If you have had a baby with spina bifida* or anencephaly*, talk with your health care provider. He or she may advise you to take even more folic acid before you get pregnant again.

Keep track of your periods

*Anencephaly:
A defect in which the brain does not develop.

It is a good idea to keep a record of your menstrual periods (monthly flow) before you get pregnant. Write the date when your period starts each month on the chart on the next page. Also count and write in the number of days of your cycle.* Knowing when your last period started will help you know when to expect your next one. This will tell you if the next one is late. It will also help you figure out when you will give birth.

*Cycle: The number of days between the start of one menstrual period and the start of the next. It is usually between 25 and 32 days long for most women.

Your doctor or nurse-midwife will need to know the date your last period started. If you do not know, she can use other methods to learn the age of your unborn baby. This will tell when your baby is likely to be born.

How do I know if I'm pregnant?

Some of the first signs of pregnancy:

- Missed menstrual period
- Tiredness
- Tender, swollen breasts
- Upset stomach

If you have two or three of these signs, you might be pregnant. Have a pregnancy test if your period is at least a week or two late. **During these early weeks, take care of yourself as if you were pregnant.**

Menstrual Period Chart
(Write dates here)

1. Date period started _____
   Month, date

2. Next period started _____
   Month, date

   Length of this cycle (number of days
   since your last period started) _____

3. Next period started _____
   Month, date

   Length of this cycle _____

4. Next period started _____
   Month, date

   Length of this cycle _____

5. Next period started _____
   Month, date

   Length of this cycle _____

A positive pregnancy test shows you are pregnant. If you have a positive test, it is time to get a physical exam. Make an appointment right away with your doctor, nurse-midwife, or clinic.

How do I get a pregnancy test?

You can buy a home pregnancy test kit at a drug store or go to your doctor or clinic. Some clinics, such as Planned Parenthood, may offer free pregnancy tests.

The home test can be done very soon after your menstrual period is late.

If a home test shows that you are **not** pregnant, wait a week or two. If your period does not come, do a second test. Then see your health care provider to find out why your period is late. If you are not pregnant, this could be a sign of other health problems.

What now?

If you are not pregnant, you have learned how to get in shape for pregnancy. If you are, you are ready to have an amazing experience in life.

Chapter 2

Now You're Pregnant— What's Next?

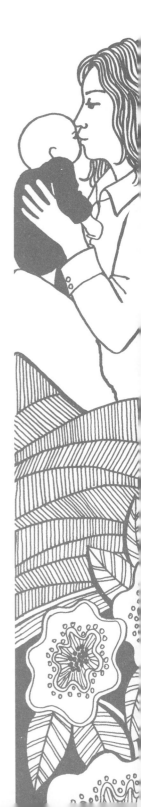

This is a time when you may feel both excited and scared. Most women have mixed feelings—and have many questions.

How will a baby change my life?

Will my baby be healthy?

What will childbirth be like?

Will I know how to be a good parent?

You will not learn the answers to all these questions right away. What you can do now is begin to live in a healthy way.

Read ahead. Chapters 3 through 6 will help you get started. Chapters 7 through 9 tell you more about the nine months of pregnancy. Look back at the end of the Introduction for a keepsake page. Here you can

---

This chapter includes:

First weeks of pregnancy, page 10
- What happens to your body
- When your baby will be born

First important steps, page 12
- Getting health care right away
- Practical things to think about

Father's or partner's role in pregnancy, page 14

write down special memories of this time. In Chapter 16 at the back of the book, you will find ideas about places to get help in your community and other ways to get more information.

Every baby is special!

If this will be your first baby, you are starting a new adventure—parenthood. If you have other children you know that every baby is one-of-a-kind and every pregnancy is different.

You might have twins or even more than two babies. This is happening more and more today. In this book we will talk mostly about a single baby, because that is most common.

What is happening to me?

Your body is starting to change in many ways. Your belly may not start to look bigger for another month or two. But you will probably begin to feel different right away.

Normal signs of pregnancy:

- Your menstrual periods have stopped. You are already about two weeks pregnant when you miss your first period!
- Your breasts may swell and become tender.
- You may feel more tired than usual.
- You may need to urinate more often than before.
- Your stomach may feel upset or you may vomit.
- You may lose a little weight.
- Your moods may change quickly. You may feel like crying one minute and be very happy the next.

How do you feel about having a baby?

✔ *Check all that you feel, or write in your thoughts:*

_____ It's wonderful.

_____ It feels strange.

_____ I can't quite believe it.

_____ I don't feel ready to have a baby.

I am a little bit afraid of _____

_____

_____

I am worried about _____

_____

_____

When will my baby be born?

A baby takes about 40 weeks to grow after the date of your last period. Your "due date" is when your baby is likely to be born. Here is how to find your due date.

Write down the date your last menstrual period started.

1. Start of your last period   _____   _____

                                                  Month   *day*

2. Add 7 days: + 7 days

3. Add 9 months: + 9 months

4. Your baby's due date: _____   _____

                                                  Month   *day*

You may not know exactly when your last period started. Your doctor or nurse practitioner can tell about when your baby is due by the:

- Size of your uterus,*

- Results of an ultrasound* test,

- Date when your baby's heartbeat is heard for the first time,

- Date when you first feel him move.

Most babies come between two weeks before and two weeks after their due dates. Be ready a few weeks before the date, in case your baby comes early.

*Uterus: The part of a woman's body where the unborn baby grows.

*Ultrasound: A way to see inside the uterus by moving a hand-held device across your belly. The test uses sound waves to make a picture of your fetus on a TV monitor.

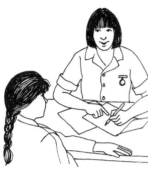

Get into care right away

You should go to a doctor, nurse practitioner, or clinic right away, so you can get the best advice for your needs. Even if you are surprised to be pregnant or are not completely ready for it, do not delay. See Chapter 5 for how to find a health care provider and to learn what your first prenatal* checkup will be like.

*Prenatal:
Before birth.

Miscarriage

It is important to know that many early pregnancies end naturally in a miscarriage.* If you have learned about your pregnancy very early, this could easily happen. You may want to wait until you reach your third or fourth month before you tell many people that you are pregnant.

*Miscarriage:
Loss of the embryo or fetus before 20 weeks, too early for a baby to survive outside the uterus (also called a "spontaneous abortion").

When miscarriage happens in the first few weeks, it usually is like a very heavy menstrual period. If you start to have light bleeding (spotting) or a heavy flow, backache, or severe cramps, call your doctor or nurse practitioner right away. (For more, see the end of Chapter 7.)

An early miscarriage usually happens when there is something wrong with the embryo or fetus or with the mother's health. These miscarriages usually cannot be stopped. You probably will feel very disappointed. Remember that most women who miscarry have no troubling having a healthy pregnancy later.

Things to consider
Paying for care

Find out how your prenatal health care and delivery will be paid for. Discuss this with your insurer, employee benefits office, or clinic. How much will be covered? What will you have to pay yourself? What choices will you have to make about care? (See Chapter 5.)

If you are a single woman

You do not have to go through this time by yourself. Good friends and family members can be wonderful support during pregnancy and birth. Find one or two people who will listen to your feelings. Take time to choose a birth partner who will be with you when your baby is born.

If you are a teenager

At this time you will be facing big changes in your life. You will have to make serious choices and new plans. You may find it hard to know what is best. Many pregnant teens face difficulties with health, money, and continuing their education.

It is important to get a pregnancy test early and start prenatal care right away. You will need to find out where to go for health care. Talk with someone you trust about your feelings. You could talk with:

- Your parents
- A nurse or advisor at school
- Your regular doctor, nurse, or community clinic
- Someone you trust at your place of worship

If you are older than age 35

There is a higher risk that older women could have health problems, compared to younger women. Also, the baby may have a greater risk of birth defects. Be sure to talk with the doctor or nurse practitioner about these risks.

If you are not sure you are ready to be a parent

Talk with a doctor, nurse, or social worker about the choices you have. Whatever you choose, be sure to take good care of your health now.

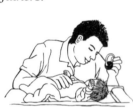

For fathers and partners

This is your pregnancy, too!

As a father-to-be, you have a special part to play. Both your wife or partner and your unborn child need your help.

Share these pages with your baby's father. Encourage him to read the book as your pregnancy goes on. There are more pages throughout the book with special notes for fathers.

The most important thing you can do is to give mother and baby your loving support. One way you can help is to learn about pregnancy. Another is to help her practice healthy habits, like stopping smoking and eating healthy foods.

You may not have learned much about being a father from your own dad. Learning more now will help you overcome many fears. Start with this book. It will give you the facts about pregnancy, delivery, and caring for a new baby.

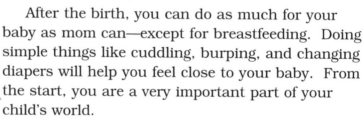

After the birth, you can do as much for your baby as mom can—except for breastfeeding. Doing simple things like cuddling, burping, and changing diapers will help you feel close to your baby. From the start, you are a very important part of your child's world.

Many fathers and partners wonder:

- Am I being left out of the excitement?
- Do my partner's moods mean she's angry with me?
- Will we still enjoy sex as pregnancy goes on and afterward?
- Will I be able to stay in the delivery room without fainting?
- Will I be a good father?

If something worries you, tell your partner about it. Talking together may help answer some of your questions. It is important for each of you to know what the other is thinking.

You also may want to talk with the doctor or nurse practitioner. Friends who are already parents can share what they have learned.

How a partner can take part in pregnancy

Here are some things you can do as a father or partner for your unborn and new baby.

Lifestyle:

• Encourage your baby's mother to eat healthy foods. Try to eat well yourself.

• Help her avoid smoking, drinking alcohol, or taking any other drugs. Find other things to do together. Plan visits with friends, listen to relaxing music, or take her for a picnic.

• If you smoke, do so outside, away from your baby's mother. Second-hand smoke affects your unborn baby and your baby later. This is a great reason for you to quit.

• Take walks and do prenatal exercises with her.

• Share home chores, like laundry, cooking, and cleaning.

Health care:

• Learn as much as you can about pregnancy and being a parent.

• Go with your partner to prenatal checkups.

• Go to childbirth classes with her. You will learn what to expect and how to help during birth.

• In the later months, put your hand on her belly. You will feel your growing baby move inside.

"It was so amazing when the ultrasound showed our baby's body moving inside. Finally I could share my partner's excitement."
— A new Dad

Feelings:

• Avoid joking or criticizing your partner's changing body shape. Many women worry about how their bodies look. Her weight gain is for her baby's health.

• Talk over your feelings about becoming parents. Let her know about your excitement and concerns. Listen to her feelings. Give her an extra hug if she is feeling unhappy.

• Talk to your baby. Unborn babies can hear voices during the last months before birth. Your baby will learn to know your voice.

Put a photo
of yourself
here

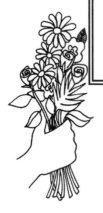

**Me,
Mother-to-Be**

Chapter 3

Staying Healthy

What you are doing every day is important for your baby's health—and your own. It is easy to say, "lead a healthy life." What does it really mean? How do you really do it?

In this chapter and the next one, you will find more about what you can do to have a healthier life and pregnancy.

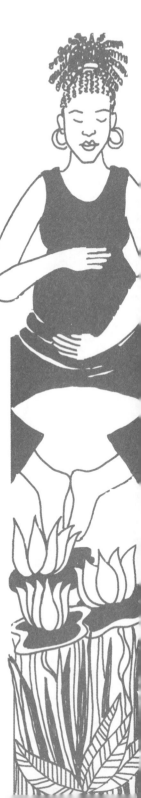

This chapter includes:

- Prenatal checkups
- Your current habits
- Learning about health

Daily living, page 22

- Teeth and gums
- Exercise
- Car safety
- Safe sex

Home and workplace, page 26

- Household hazards
- Risks at work

Mental Health, page 28

- Stress and relaxation
- Spouse or partner abuse

Keys to Good Health During Pregnancy

These healthy habits apply to everyone, woman or man, young or old. However, they have special meaning for you and your unborn baby. Some may not seem to affect pregnancy, such as tooth brushing. However, in this chapter and the next you will find out how important they are to you now.

- Go to all your health checkups.
- Avoid alcohol, cigarettes, second-hand smoke, and drugs.
- Eat healthy foods.
- Buckle your safety belt every time you ride in a car, truck, or van.
- Exercise regularly.
- Learn to relax and accept all your feelings.
- Brush and floss your teeth daily.
- Protect yourself from disease during sex.

If I'm feeling fine, why do I need prenatal checkups?

"Prenatal care" is health care during pregnancy. You will have a number of prenatal checkups. These help your doctor or nurse-midwife know how you and your baby are changing and what your needs are. She will look for health problems that you may not notice, like high blood pressure.

If your health is good, you will have one checkup each month. In the last two months before birth, you will be checked more often.

Your health care provider will check:

- your baby's growth, heart rate, and movement;
- how you feel and how your body is changing;
- your weight gain and food habits;
- your blood pressure* and urine for signs of health problems; other tests will be done, too, to see how the baby is growing;

*Blood pressure: The force of the blood pumped by the heart through your blood vessels. High blood pressure means the heart is working extra hard.

The chances are good that you will have no serious problems. But a serious problem is easier to treat if it is found early.

Your doctor or nurse-midwife wants to hear your concerns. The checkup is your best time to ask questions. As you go through this book, write down questions that you want to ask.

For more about checkups and finding a provider, see Chapter 5.

Learning about health

There is a lot to learn. You are making a good start by using this book. You will read and hear all kinds of advice from friends, family, TV, newspapers, and the Internet. Some information can be very confusing. A product or activity that you are told is healthy one day may be found to be unhealthy the next day.

Here are some questions to ask before you trust something new that you hear or read:

- What is the original source (person, company, or organization) of the information? Is it a source that you can trust, such as a well-known national medical organization?

- Does the source make money from the new information? Is it selling something?

- Is the report new or old?

- How does the information compare with what other sources say (including your own doctor or nurse)?

Introducing your unborn baby

Here are life-sized pictures showing the growth of an unborn baby in the first four months. See how quickly a baby grows and changes (develops)! All the main parts of the body (brain, spinal cord, and organs) are formed very early. This is why you need to take care of yourself during this time.

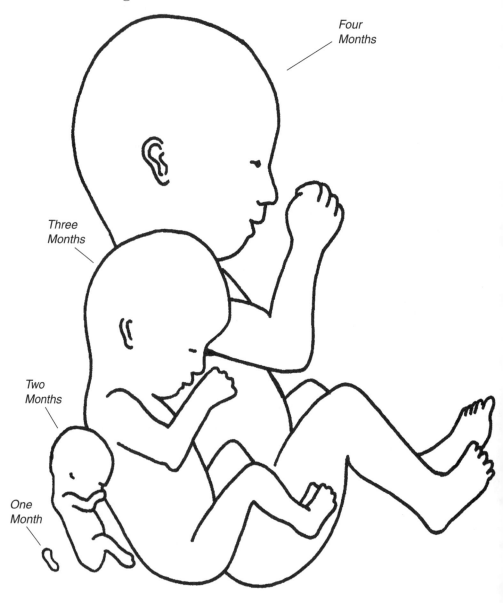

Four Months

Three Months

Two Months

One Month

How your baby grows
(Life-size pictures)

How healthy are your habits?

Most of us already have some habits that help an unborn baby. Some of our other habits could be unhealthy. Check your healthy habits on the list below. Be honest with yourself—for the health of your baby!

Yes	No	Healthy Habits
❏	❏	I eat five or more servings of fruits and vegetables daily.
❏	❏	I drink at least eight glasses of water and other liquids every day.
❏	❏	I do not smoke.
❏	❏	I do not drink beer, wine, wine coolers, or hard liquor now.
❏	❏	I do not take drugs, except those my doctor has prescribed.
❏	❏	I get about seven to eight hours of sleep every night.
❏	❏	I exercise for about 30 minutes at least three times a week.
❏	❏	I take some time to relax every day.
❏	❏	I talk over my worries with others.
❏	❏	I brush my teeth and floss daily.

Did you answer "no" to any questions above?
Those are the most important things for you to try to change while you are pregnant.

Write down the habits that you want to change:

_____

_____

_____

_____

Nobody's perfect, but you are making a good start!

You may need help in making these changes. Talk with your doctor, nurse-midwife, your partner, or another person you trust.

Care of your teeth and gums

Here is some information that may surprise you. It is based on sound research. The health of your mouth is important during pregnancy. The germs that cause gum disease can make your body go into labor too early. (These germs also can harm people who are not pregnant. They have an effect on heart disease, diabetes, and other illnesses.)

Brushing and flossing is usually enough to prevent gum disease, but you also need regular checkups by your dentist. If your gums are red and swollen or bleed easily, you may have gum disease. Be sure to have your dentist treat the disease.

Keep Moving

Why should I exercise?

Some of the best reasons to exercise are:

- Exercise keeps your blood flowing well. This keeps your legs from swelling. It may help prevent bulging blue veins (varicose veins) in your legs or hemorrhoids.*

*Hemorrhoids: Bulging veins in your anus (where bowel movements come out) that may ache or itch.

- It may help prevent illness by strengthening your immune system to fight disease.

- It relaxes your mind as well as your muscles. It can help you sleep better.

- It helps you have regular bowel movements.

- It can prevent or lessen backaches.

How to exercise during pregnancy

Talk with your doctor or nurse-midwife about the kinds of exercise you are doing or want to start doing.

- Walking is one of the best exercises for anyone. It is also one of the easiest and costs nothing. The only equipment you need is a pair of flat, cushioned sport shoes. Walk for about a half-hour on most days if possible. Start slowly and then walk fast enough to sweat a little bit.

- If you have not been exercising, do something easy like walking. (See pages 95 and 96 for some other specific exercises.)

- You can usually continue the kind of exercise you were doing before your pregnancy. Avoid high-impact aerobics and risky sports.

- Exercise at least three or four times each week for real benefits.

- Drink plenty of water before and afterward. Try not to get overheated. Stop if you feel dizzy or faint. Exercise when the weather is cool.

- It may be easier to exercise with a friend than alone. You can encourage each other.

"My friend and I decided to walk together once a week. We need each other to push us to actually get out the door. This way we have a chance to catch up on all the latest gossip, too."

Buckle up for two

Car travel seems so safe, but driving to the grocery store, mall, or your job may be the most dangerous thing you do. It also is the biggest danger to your unborn child.

Crashes are the most common cause of death and injury to young men and women. If you are hurt in a car, van, or truck crash, your unborn baby may be hurt, too. The uterus cannot cushion your baby from the forces of a car crash. Even if you are not injured, your baby could be harmed.

Safe riding:

Protect yourself from injury:

- Use the lap-shoulder belt (and using a car with air bags, if possible).

- Sit in the back seat when you can. It is safer than the front seat for everyone.

- Say "no" to riding with a driver who has been drinking or using drugs.

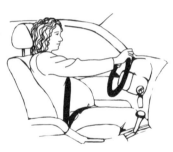

Protect your baby:

- Keep the lap belt under your belly.

- Wear the shoulder belt across the middle of your shoulder.

- Drive as little as possible in the last few months. Let someone else drive, so you are not sitting behind the steering wheel.

Wearing safety belts correctly

- **Use both the lap and shoulder belts.** The shoulder belt greatly increases your safety. It keeps your head from hitting the windshield or dashboard or other parts of the car. It also keeps your body from folding forward and pressing on your uterus. If your car has separate lap and shoulder belts, be sure to buckle both of them.

- **Push the lap belt down under your belly, touching your thighs.** Make the lap belt snug. The lap belt must be below your uterus so it will not press on your uterus in a crash.

Air bag safety

The frontal air bags are in the steering wheel and dashboard. They do not take the place of safety belts. They work with the belt to protect your head and chest in front-end crashes. Your safety belt holds you in place during rollovers and rear-end or side crashes.

Frontal air bags work best if you sit as far back from them as possible. Slide your seat back to allow plenty of space for the air bag to open.

The air bag will not harm your fetus. However, if you are very short and have to drive yourself, it is important to sit as far back as possible (10 inches, if possible) from the center of the steering wheel. Try reclining your seat back and driving with your arms straight. Tilt the steering wheel to face your chest.

If your car has side air bags,* try not to lean against the door while riding. Check the vehicle owner's manual for advice.

*Side air bag: A small air bag that comes out of the door, the side of the seat, or above the door. It reduces injuries from a crash into the side of your vehicle.

If you are in a crash

If you are in a car crash, get yourself checked at the emergency room or doctor's office right away. Be sure to tell the doctor you are pregnant.

A serious injury could happen even if you do not think you have been hurt. Your fetus, the uterus, or the placenta could be hurt even if you used a safety belt and the air bag inflated.

Baby needs a car seat

After your baby is born, he or she will need a car seat (child safety seat). These seats protect babies very well and are required by law in all states. (See Chapter 6 for details.)

Safe sex

While you are pregnant, it is nice not to have to think about birth control. However, if you are not in a sexual relationship with only one person, it is very important to protect yourself from diseases that spread through sex (sexually transmitted diseases or STDs).

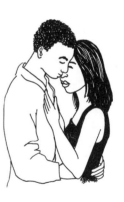

Herpes, chlamydia, syphilis, gonorrhea, hepatitis B, and HIV/AIDS are all STDs. Any of these diseases could harm your unborn baby as well as you.

Your doctor or nurse-midwife will test you for some of these diseases at your first checkup. If you think that you may have an STD, be sure to tell your provider. There are cures for most STDs.

Most STDs can be treated, so your baby can be born healthy.

HIV-AIDS is the most serious STD because it has no cure. However, treatment can keep it from spreading from mother to unborn baby. An HIV test is important for every pregnant woman, because many women do not know they have HIV.

Preventing STDs

Not getting an STD is much better for your health than curing one. Three ways to prevent STDs are:

1. Have one faithful sex partner for many years.

2. Do not have sex at all.

3. Use a condom and a spermicide,* every time you have sex. This is not as safe as the first two suggestions.

Hazards around the house

Cat litter boxes

Cat feces* may have parasites that could infect you and your unborn baby. They can cause birth defects. You may not feel sick, but your baby could be harmed.

Any kitten or cat that goes outdoors could catch these parasites. Ask someone else to clean the litter box while you are pregnant. If you work in a garden where cat feces may be, wear gloves.

Lead in the air, soil, and water

Lead is a poisonous metal that may cause miscarriage or brain damage to unborn babies and children. Lead can be found in household dust, air, and water and in soil near highways. It also is found in factories where painting or soldering is done.

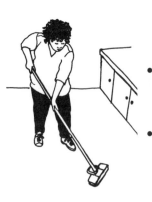

- Do you work with lead? Ask for another job while you are pregnant or breastfeeding. If someone else in your household works with lead, make sure they take off work clothes and shoes before coming home.

- Lead can be in dirt around homes or on shoes or clothes from a factory. Mop floors frequently. Make sure children wash hands after playing outside.

- Paint used in older homes and on furniture before 1978 was made with lead. People may breathe paint dust or eat tiny chips of paint without knowing it. Even a very small amount can harm a fetus or small child.

*Spermicide: A cream or jelly used with a condom to kill germs as well as sperm that could be passed during sex.

*Feces: Bowel movements.

It is important to cover the old paint with new paint. When repainting an older home, a pregnant woman and any children should move out to avoid paint dust.

- Lead in the pipes of old houses may get into the water. Avoid drinking the water that has been sitting in the pipes overnight. Run the water for a few minutes in the morning before using it. Hot water absorbs more lead than cold water. When cooking and making coffee or tea, start with cold water from the tap.

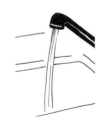

- Young children living in areas with lead in old homes or in the soil should be tested by the doctor.

Hot tubs and saunas

It is best not to use a hot tub or sauna while you are pregnant. The very hot water or air might harm your baby by raising your body temperature.

Could my work affect my baby?

This depends on the kind of job you have and how well you are feeling. Some problems during pregnancy could be made worse by your work. Some jobs could cause health problems. What you can do about it depends on the company you work for.

If you have a desk job, you may not have job-related health problems. However, it is important to get up and walk around during the day. Take a walk outside during your lunch break at least.

Do you face dangers in your job? Are there toxic chemicals or lead in your area? Do you work around X-rays, such as in a dentist's office? All these things could cause problems in pregnancy. Ask to work away from such dangers if you can.

Does your job give your body a lot of stress? Do you have to sit or stand all day? Do you have shift changes that make it hard to get enough sleep? Do you have to lift and carry heavy things? Are you required to work extra-long hours? These things may help:

*Support stockings: Elastic stockings (hose) that fit very snugly around your legs to reduce swelling and help prevent varicose veins.

- Wear flat shoes and support stockings.*
- Do exercises like the pelvic tilt (page 95) to strengthen your back.
- Ask for rest times to walk around or put your feet up.

Talk to your doctor and your employer if you think your health could be in danger. Ask your company to give you another task while you are pregnant. If you are having health problems, you may be able to get a leave of absence or disability leave.

Learn to relax and reduce stress

How you think and feel affects your body. Keeping your mind free of stress helps you stay healthy. It may even help you get better if you are sick. Enjoying little things in life, like having a good laugh over a joke, can make the hard parts easier.

Some things about being pregnant may not be pleasant. You may have aches and pains. Pregnancy may add extra stress to your family or job.

Some things may be both exciting and scary, like thinking about raising your child. Others can give you joy. Feeling your unborn baby kick you in the ribs can be a thrill!

Help yourself to feel more content

You can learn ways to relax. This will help you find your own way to cope with the difficulties of pregnancy. Some things you could do for yourself are:

- Take a nap or spend some time reading.
- Rest your hand on your belly and feel your baby moving.
- Talk to your unborn child.
- Learn to knit or sew so you can make a baby blanket or quilt.
- Watch funny movies that make you laugh a lot.

- Take a warm shower.
- Talk with friends.
- Exercise.

How can other people help me?

We all live with others—in small families or large ones, with school friends, work friends, and neighbors. These people are your support system. They can help in many ways now and after your baby comes.

Your husband or partner can share your joy and your worries. Your parents, brothers and sisters, other relatives, and friends also can give you support and comfort.

Be sure to tell your doctor or nurse-midwife about any problems in your life. Changes in your job, a move to a new town, or family problems can give you a lot of stress. Your health care provider needs to know about your stress.

Remember: Both parents feel stress. Your baby's father may need extra hugs and time to relax, too. You are in this together.

Telling people what you need

You may know that all these people care. But they may not know what they can do to help you. Try to tell them what you want, like this:

- "Today I am very tired. Could you please care for my little boy, so I can take a nap?"
- "Let's watch a funny movie, not a sad one."
- "Please help with the laundry. My back aches."

Trouble at home?

Help for abused women

Some women's husbands or partners may hit, kick, beat, or shout at them. This abuse often begins or gets worse during pregnancy. Children in the family also might be attacked. **Domestic violence is a crime. It**

also is a serious health problem that harms both mother, unborn baby, and other children in the home.

If this is happening to you, you are not to blame. The person who attacks you is the one who is doing something wrong. Even if the attacker only shouts and calls you names, that can hurt you.

If you are being abused, you do not need to take it!

Getting help

- Call a crisis hotline. There is a free National Domestic Violence Hotline, 800-799-7233. It can give you information and local contacts for shelters, counseling, and legal help.

- Tell a trusted friend, doctor or nurse, clergy member, or mental health counselor.

- Find out where to get help in the community, such as a legal aid program or a counselor.

- Learn about safe places to go if you need to leave. A battered women's shelter can give you protection.

Being a good friend

Do you know another woman who fears her husband or partner? Tell her of your concern and support her in getting help. Share the free hotline number above.

Women often hide signs of abuse. Some signs to look for are:

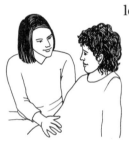

- Bruises or other injuries blamed on "accidents"

- Staying home alone most of the time

- Increased alcohol or drug use

Chapter 4

What You Eat, Drink, and Breathe

Almost everything you take into your body can affect your baby's growth and health. Many things you eat, drink, and breathe pass through the placenta and into your baby's blood. Being good to your own body is important for both of you. It even is important to think about the air you breathe.

Some kinds of foods, drinks, and drugs can harm a growing fetus. You are the only one who can make sure your unborn baby is not exposed to these substances. It can be hard to change habits but that can make a big difference to your baby.

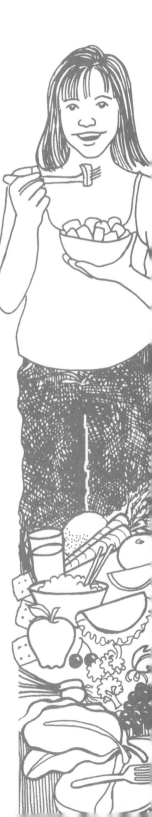

This chapter includes:

Healthy eating, page 32

- Healthy eating and exercise
- Prenatal vitamins

Things that can harm your baby, page 38

- Food warnings and safety
- Medicines, herbs
- Alcohol, tobacco, and drugs
- How to stop smoking

Smart eating for baby and you

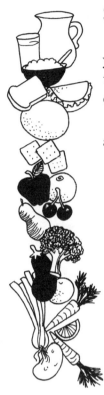

Nutritious foods help your body stay strong and your baby's body and brain develop well. Eating well takes some planning. You may have to change some of your habits.

Try different foods to find things you like that are also healthy for you:

- List the foods you usually eat now. Compare them to the healthiest foods listed on the next page.

- Make an effort to eat more of the healthy foods and less of the others.

- Try a new food each week.

- Make a list of healthy foods before you go to the grocery store. Make sure to have at least some of them in the kitchen at all times.

- Eat some foods that are not your favorites. Do this for your baby. You may grow to like them.

- Remember that exercise goes along with healthy eating.

Seven nutrients* your body needs

*Nutrients:
Vitamins, minerals, and other things in food that everyone needs for health and to help a fetus grow.

1. **Protein**—for growth of muscles, organs, and cells.

2. **Carbohydrates**—for energy.

3. **Fats**—for energy and cell growth.

4. **Vitamins**—for making the organs, muscles, nerves, and other parts of your body work right.

5. **Minerals**—for healthy growth of cells in bones, teeth, and blood.

6. **Fiber**—for better digestion of foods and prevention of certain diseases.

7. **Water**—for normal working of the entire body. All parts of your body contain a lot of water.

If you are under age 18, you need extra protein and foods with calcium, like cheese and milk. This is because your own body is still growing. These foods build your bones and muscles as well as your baby's body.

The healthiest foods—examples

Here are examples of the kinds of foods that give you the most and best nutrients. Try to eat a wide variety of foods. These foods are best for everyone, not just pregnant women.

How many of these do you eat every day?

- **Vegetables** (3 to 5 servings)
  Broccoli, squash, sweet potatoes, tomatoes, spinach, collard greens, and bok choy—dark green or bright colored vegetables are best.

- **Fruits** (2 to 3 servings)
  Oranges, papaya, apples, melons, prunes, and raisins—bright colored fruits are best.

- **Breads and other whole grains** (with every meal)
  Wheat bread, corn tortillas, brown rice, rye crackers, and cooked or dry whole-grain cereal. Eat whole grains. They have much more taste and nutrients than white bread, white rice, or spaghetti.

- **Dairy and other calcium-rich foods** (3 to 4 servings)
  Non-fat or low-fat milk, hard cheese, cottage cheese, and yogurt, tofu made with calcium (check the label), calcium tablets (supplements). If milk makes you feel ill, eat other calcium-rich foods (see page 36).

- **Fish, poultry, eggs** (1 to 2 servings)
  Salmon, catfish, snapper, chicken, turkey, and eggs (beware of some fish, see page 39).

- **Beans and nuts** (1 to 3 servings)
  Lentils, garbanzo beans, black-eyed peas, walnuts, almonds, peanuts, and tofu.

- **Oils** (have a small amount at all meals)
  Plant oils from corn, safflower, canola, olives, or peanuts (in cooking, in salad dressings, and with bread).

- **Water and other liquids** (8 tall glasses)
  Water is best, along with milk, fruit or vegatable juice (100 percent juice), soup, and a cup or two of coffee and tea. (Avoid regular or diet sodas, power drinks, and sugary juice drinks.)

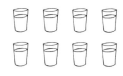

- **Foods to limit** (have only as treats)
  Red meat, butter, sweets and sodas, white bread, pasta, and white potatoes. (These have few nutrients. They take the place of nutritious foods and can lead to illness.)

Most people eat too much fat and sugar in processed foods, fast foods, and snack foods. Learn to enjoy the taste of whole grain breads and fresh vegetables. You will be healthier and you often will save money, too.

How big is a serving?

A small bowl of food for one person may seem like a huge meal to another. Experts who plan healthy diets suggest servings that are smaller than many people realize.

More is not better. Many restaurants serve large amounts, much more than one serving. Products like cookies, muffins, and soft drinks often come in large sizes. These have many more calories, fats, and sugar than is healthy.

Try measuring foods to see how big a serving is. Read the labels on packages, too.

Examples of serving sizes:

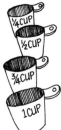

Fruit: 1 medium orange, 1/2 cup applesauce, 3/4 cup juice

Vegetables: 1 cup raw lettuce, 1/2 cup cooked squash, 3/4 cup juice

Grains: 1 slice of whole wheat bread, 1/2 cup brown rice, 1 ounce (1/2 to 1 cup) dry cereal

Meats and beans: 2 to 3 ounces meat, poultry or fish (the size of a pack of cards), two eggs, 1 cup cooked kidney beans or lentils

Dairy foods: 1 cup milk or yogurt, 1 1/2 ounces (a slice) cheddar cheese, 2 cups cottage cheese

Other: 1 tablespoon olive oil, salad dressing, catsup, or jelly

Six healthy eating habits

Now is a good time to begin eating better for your whole family's health. The foods you should eat during pregnancy are good for your lifetime.

1. Choose brightly colored vegetables and fruits as major parts of meals and snacks. Remember "Five-a-day," the slogan for eating enough fruits and vegetables.

2. Use whole grain cereals and breads.

3. Serve fish, chicken, or turkey instead of hamburger, ribs, or bologna. Try some meals with tofu or dry beans.

4. Choose low-fat or non-fat (skim) milk, yogurt, cottage cheese, and frozen yogurt.

5. Cook with liquid oils, like olive, peanut, corn, and soybean oil, instead of butter, lard, or coconut oil.

6. Eat less fried food, take smaller servings of salad dressing, use olive oil instead of butter on your bread.

"When I'm shopping for groceries, I try to make sure I have a variety of foods in my cart. That helps me make meals that aren't boring.

Eating out, eating wisely

Restaurant meals are often loaded with fats and lacking in the nutritious foods you and your baby need. If you eat out often, choose the places and the menu items that will be best for you. Look for:

- a salad bar where you can mix your own spinach, tomatoes, kidney beans, peppers, and mushrooms

- salad dressing "on the side" so you can add as little as you want

Super-sized burgers and sodas aren't bargains. They can be hazardous to your health.

- main dishes of fish or chicken, broiled or baked—not fried or covered with thick sauce or gravy

- foods that are not too oily or salty

Many restaurants advertise huge servings—more than is healthy for anyone. You could share a main course with a friend. If you want dessert, try sharing it, too. This saves money and cuts down on the extra calories you don't need.

If you are a vegetarian

A vegetarian can eat most of the foods listed earlier. To get enough protein during pregnancy, you will need to eat a variety of dry beans and peas, tofu, nuts, eggs, and dairy products.

If you do not eat dairy products and eggs, you will need to be extra careful to get enough protein and calcium. Be sure to talk to your health care provider about how to get all the nutrients you need now.

Getting enough calcium

While you are pregnant, you need to eat plenty of calcium. Calcium makes your baby's bones and teeth strong. It also keeps your bones strong.

Milk has much more calcium than most foods. But some adults find that milk gives them gas, cramps, and diarrhea.* This is called "lactose intolerance." It is very common among adults who are African-American, Hispanic, Asian-American, and Native-American. **Tell your doctor or nurse-midwife if milk makes you feel sick.**

*Diarrhea (Die-a-ree-a): Bowel movements that come more often than normal and are very soft and watery.

If you have lactose intolerance, you may be able to eat some foods made from milk. Try yogurt with live cultures, or hard cheese like cheddar or Swiss. You may find "low lactose" milk and milk custard or pudding easier to eat. Your health care provider may suggest lactaid or calcium supplements, such as Tums.

Some foods also give you calcium, but you need to eat a lot of them to get enough. These are:

- collard greens, kale, cabbage, radishes, bok choy, parsnips, broccoli,
- orange juice with calcium added
- canned salmon or sardines with bones
- tofu made with "calcium sulfate" (see the label)
- corn tortillas made with lime
- black-eyed peas and other dry beans; sesame seeds, almonds, and peanuts
- blackstrap molasses

Prenatal vitamins every day

While you are pregnant, it is very important to get enough of the right vitamins. It is very hard to get all the vitamins you need from your food. You can be sure you are getting enough by taking a prenatal vitamin pill every day. If you don't like to take big pills, you can cut them in half, but take both pieces in one day.

Choose a multi-vitamin that has 100 percent of vitamins and minerals. Check the label. It is important not to take **more** than the recommended amount of vitamins daily, so cut out other vitamin supplements. (Multi-vitamin pills do not contain the full amount of calcium, so you can take a calcium supplement.)

Iron is found in most prenatal vitamins. It is a very important mineral for you during pregnancy. It is hard to get enough iron in your food.

Some women worry that iron may make them constipated. It is best not to cut out iron because of constipation. There are other ways to prevent constipation. You can eat foods such as whole grains, bran cereal, and fruits (especially prunes) every day. Drink plenty of water. If you still have a problem, talk to your doctor or nurse.

A vitamin pill does not take the place of eating a wide variety of healthy foods.

Folic Acid

One of the most important vitamins during pregnancy is folic acid (also called folate). In the first few weeks, it helps prevent very serious defects in the baby's spinal column and brain (see Chapter 1). It continues to be important for your baby's growth all during pregnancy. You should have at least 400 mcg daily. Many doctors advise even more (600 mcg) while you are pregnant.

Prenatal vitamins have at least 400 mcg of folic acid. You can get some from eating foods like dark green, leafy vegetables, orange juice, dry cereals, breads, and pasta. However, it is very hard to get enough from foods alone.

Vitamin A: Too much of a good thing?

Vitamin A is very important for health, but too much can cause birth defects. You will get enough in a prenatal vitamin (up to 5,000 IU) and in green and yellow vegetables you eat. Do not take extra vitamin supplements or eat liver. Liver has too much vitamin A for a pregnant woman.

Coffee, tea, and soft drinks

Coffee and tea have caffeine in them. Small amounts are not harmful. **But, when coffee makes you feel jumpy, your baby gets that way, too.** A large amount of coffee (5 or more cups) per day seems to increase the risk of miscarriage. Caffeine also limits the vitamins and minerals a woman gets from food. If you like these drinks, limit how much you drink.

Caffeine is found in many cold medicines, diet pills, and headache pills. Some is found in many soft drinks like Coca-Cola, Pepsi, Mountain Dew, Dr. Pepper, and sport drinks. Read the labels before using these things.

Food warnings

- **Salty foods:** Everyone needs a little salt every day, but too much is not healthy. You can eat some salt unless you have certain problems with your health, such as high blood pressure. Ask your health care provider if you need to limit salt.

Be aware that some foods, like chips, pickles, fast foods, and pre-made foods, have much larger amounts of salt than anyone needs. Look on the label for the amount of sodium. Salt is even in some things that do not taste salty.

- **Eating things that are not foods, like dirt, clay, ice, or laundry starch:** Some women like to eat such things when they are pregnant. This is called pica. These substances can take the place of the foods your body needs, so it is best to limit this kind of eating. These things do not give you the nutrition your baby needs to develop well.

  If you crave such non-foods, it is important to tell your doctor or nurse-midwife. Pica could give you health problems or may be a sign of a problem.

- **Food supplements:** Some food supplements could be harmful during pregnancy. They are not tested for safety during pregnancy, so it is best to not use them. Ask your doctor or nurse-midwife before using them.

- **Danger of mercury in some fish:** Fish are very nutritious, but a few kinds contain a lot of mercury. Mercury is a poison that can harm the brains of unborn babies and young children. While you are pregnant or nursing or have young children, it is very important to eat only the right kinds of fish.

  Do not eat these fish:

  - Shark, swordfish, king mackerel, and tilefish: eat none.

  - Fresh-water fish caught by family or friends: eat no more than one small serving (6 ounces) per week. This varies in different rivers, lakes, and ocean areas. Check with your local health department or fishing regulation booklet.

Fish you can eat safely include: farmed trout or catfish, shrimp, "fish sticks," flounder, salmon, haddock, and "light" canned tuna (not white tuna). You and your young children can eat two servings of fish each week safely. If you have more one week, eat less the following week.

Learn about WIC

The **Women, Infants, and Children Program** called "WIC" is an excellent national program. It is not just for very low-income families. Many pregnant women qualify to use it for nutritious foods. WIC also gives helpful prenatal and infant care information. Call 800-942-9467 to find how to reach your local WIC program.

Food Safety

People often get sick from food that is not clean or that has spoiled from being stored unsafely. Follow these general rules:

- Wash your hands well before handling food and before eating.

- Cook raw or undercooked meat, poultry, fish, eggs, or shellfish (clams and oysters) well. They may have bacteria in them (see Listeriosis, below).

- Keep raw meat away from vegetables and fruits you plan to eat uncooked.

- After handling raw meats, wash your hands with soap and hot water. Scrub the cutting board well, too.

- Eat prepared foods very soon after buying them (foods like roast chicken, salads, pizza, and sandwiches).

- Wash fruits and vegetables well before eating.

- Keep your refrigerator cold (under 40 degrees).

- Keep leftovers no more than a few days.

Listeriosis—a serious food hazard

Listeriosis is a very serious illness for a pregnant woman. You can get it from undercooked or unclean foods. It can cause miscarriage, preterm labor, or death to a newborn baby.

Pregnant women, small children, elderly people, and others with certain diseases should:

- Cook all meats, poultry, and fish well. Canned fish and packaged seafood can be eaten safely.

- Eat prepared meats (hotdogs, lunch meats) only if you heat them to steaming hot.

- Stay away from soft cheeses like feta, Camembert, Mexican-style cheese, cheese with blue veins. Hard and semi-soft cheese (such as cheddar and mozzarella), cream cheese, and cottage cheese do not carry listeria.

- Avoid raw (unpasteurized) milk or foods made with it.

Things that can harm your baby

Almost anything you eat, drink, or breathe will reach your baby in the uterus. Healthy food and fresh air are the substances your baby needs. Keep your baby safe from medicines, alcohol, tobacco, and drugs.

How often do you take an aspirin pill or a spoonful of cough medicine? When was the last time you had too many cups of coffee or sat in a smoky room? Do you ever use food supplements and herbs instead of regular medicines? Do you like to have wine or beer with dinner?

If you are pregnant, any of these might harm your baby. Remember that your unborn child is much smaller than you are. Even a very small amount of some things could do harm.

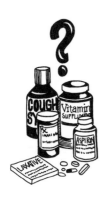

Medicines

Check with your doctor or nurse-midwife before taking any medicines, supplements, or herbs, including:

- Medicines prescribed by a doctor before you were pregnant
- Aspirin, vitamin pills, laxatives, cold medicines, and herbal medicines you can buy without a prescription

Alcohol, tobacco, and drugs = Babies in danger

Some drugs, especially alcohol, tobacco, and most street drugs, could cause very serious health effects both to you and your baby. **If you find that you cannot stop using any of these things, now is the time to get help.**

It is important for your health care provider to know about any drugs you may use. Try to be honest with her. She will know where you can get treatment.

How does alcohol harm babies?

Of course, no mother would try to harm her unborn baby. However, if you drink beer, wine, or mixed drinks, the alcohol goes from your blood stream into your baby's body.

Alcohol can hurt the brain before birth. It can slow the unborn baby's growth and give him other problems. Children harmed by alcohol may have problems with health, learning, and behavior as they grow up. This is called Fetal Alcohol Syndrome.*

Serious harm can be done when the baby is just starting to grow. That is why it is important to stop drinking as soon as you think you might be pregnant. Alcohol can affect your baby's development all through pregnancy. It can harm a baby who is breastfeeding, too.

*Fetal Alcohol Syndrome: The severe health and developmental problems of a child who has been damaged by alcohol before birth. It includes both mental retardation and physical defects. Also called "FAS."

No one knows how much a woman can drink safely, so it is safest not to drink at all. Even a little alcohol might harm a baby to some degree. You do not have to be an alcoholic to have a child affected by alcohol.

Facts about alcohol

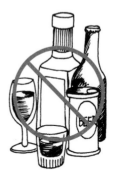

- Fetal Alcohol Syndrome is the most preventable kind of mental retardation.

- A woman's blood absorbs more alcohol from a drink than a man's body does. This means the same size drink will affect you more than a man. The alcohol in your blood will affect your baby.

- There is about the same amount of alcohol in a can of beer, a bottle of wine cooler, a glass of wine, and a shot of hard liquor.

- "Coolers" and many mixed drinks taste like soft drinks. They often have a lot of alcohol in them, however.

Is it hard to quit drinking?

If you are not able to stop drinking easily, you will need help. Talk with your family about your effort to stop. Your doctor or nurse-midwife can help you get counseling. It may be hard to quit, but it will be best for both you and your baby.

Tips to make quitting easier:

- Stay out of places where people are drinking.

- If others in your family drink, let them know why you are trying not to drink. Ask them to do other things with you. You could get some exercise or cook a nice dinner together.

- If you feel like drinking when you are alone, find something else to do. Go see a friend who does not drink, take a walk, or see a movie.

This important time in your life is also the best time to quit drinking!

Drinking and driving can hurt too!

Both you and your baby could be hurt if you drink and drive. Riding with someone who has been drinking is also very risky. In a crash you and your unborn baby could easily be harmed.

If your driver has been drinking, stay safe by:

- Driving yourself, or
- Taking a cab home, or
- Asking for a ride with someone who has not been drinking, or
- Staying with friends.

Be sure to buckle your lap-shoulder belt whenever you are in a moving vehicle.

How does smoking harm babies?

Your baby needs the oxygen in clean air. That oxygen passes into his body through your blood. Your blood also carries carbon monoxide,* nicotine,* and other chemicals from cigarettes to your unborn baby. Nicotine makes his heart beat faster. Carbon monoxide takes the place of oxygen in his blood.

*Carbon Monoxide: A poisonous gas that results from burning tobacco or other things.

*Nicotine: A chemical in tobacco that is very harmful.

Smoking could cause a miscarriage or preterm birth. Babies of smokers often are born smaller than other babies because they get less oxygen. After birth, they also may have problems, such as more colds, lung illness, and ear infections than other children.

Second-hand smoke

Smoke from other peoples' cigarettes affects your health. It also reaches your baby in the uterus and can cause harm. If your friends smoke, ask them not to smoke in your home. And stay out of smoky places.

Quitting smoking

This is one of the most important things you can do for your baby's health. Even if you quit in the middle of pregnancy, you are helping your baby.

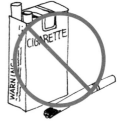

Ask your doctor or nurse-midwife for help quitting. Talk to him about using a nicotine patch or gum. Also ask your partner and friends to support you while you quit.

Here are some things to think about:

- Why I want to stop (ideas: "for my baby's health," or "it is too expensive."):

  _____

  _____

- Things I can do when I feel like smoking (ideas: "have a mint after eating" or "not hang out with people who smoke."):

  _____

  _____

- I will save this much money in a week by not buying cigarettes: $_____*

- Things I can do with the money I'll save (ideas: "hire a babysitter so I can go to the movies" or "start a savings account for my baby"):

  _____

  _____

*To find how much you're saving, multiply the price per pack by the number of packs per day by 7 days

- What to say if someone starts smoking near me (ideas: "please go outside to smoke" or "please don't—it might make me start again"):

  _____

  _____

- Set a quitting date in the next two weeks and write it down: _____.

- Here are things I'll do on that day (ideas: "flush all my cigarettes down the toilet" and "tell my friends and family and ask for their help"):

  _____

  _____

On quitting day

Get rid of all your cigarettes and ashtrays in your home, car, and workplace. Tell all your friends you have quit and ask for their help.

Take good care of yourself by taking a long walk or going out with non-smoking friends. Every time you want a cigarette, distract yourself with gum or a toothpick to chew on. The feeling will last only a few minutes.

You will probably start feeling better in about two or three weeks. If you start smoking again, know that you have not failed. Throw out the cigarettes and try again.

Illegal drugs

Illegal drugs, like cocaine, heroin, PCP, methamphetamine, and others, can be very dangerous for unborn babies. When a pregnant woman gets high, her unborn baby does, too. What might make you feel good for a short time may do life-long harm to your child.

Using these drugs even a few times could harm an unborn child. If you have a drug habit, now is the time to get help and quit. It may not be easy, but having a healthy baby is worth it!

Drugs can cause:

- An early miscarriage
- Heavy bleeding late in pregnancy
- Early delivery, which can cause other problems
- A baby born addicted who must go through the pain of withdrawal
- A child who has trouble learning or behaving as other children do

The sooner you can stop smoking, drinking, or taking drugs, the better for both of you. This can be hard to do, but you can do it.

Chapter 5

Medical Care During Pregnancy and Childbirth

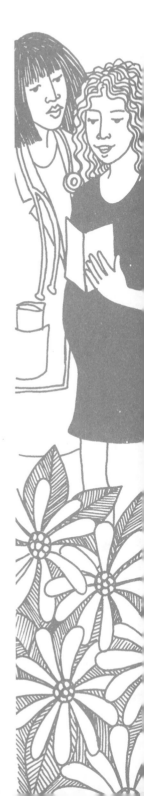

It is important to have a checkup at least once a month while you are pregnant. Even when you are feeling well, you should see a health care provider (doctor or nurse-midwife) regularly. These visits will help you stay healthy and deal with any problems early.

Every pregnant woman needs to choose a heath care provider and a place to give birth. Your choices depend on where you live and on your health insurance plan, if you have one. Most plans have a list of hospitals and providers that you can use. You may be able to use the family doctor you already go to.

If you are not sure where to go for care, call:

- your insurance benefits office
- local public health department
- community clinic
- nearby hospital

This chapter includes:

Where your baby will be born, page 48

- How to choose a doctor or nurse practitioner

What to expect at prenatal checkups, page 51

- Using medical services wisely

Choosing a doctor for your baby, page 53

Paying for care

Find out how your prenatal health care and delivery will be paid for. Discuss this with your insurer, employee benefits office, or clinic. What kinds of services are paid for by your plan? How much will be covered? How much will you have to pay yourself? What choices will you have to make about care?

If you do not have health insurance, find out about options from your local health department. You may qualify for state insurance. There also are community health centers that base their fees on your income (a sliding-fee scale). Look ahead to care for your baby. Ask about the Children's Health Insurance Program (CHIP).

Where will my baby be born?

Many women want to give birth at a particular kind of place. In some areas, there are choices of hospitals, birth centers in hospitals, and separate birth centers. Some midwives may offer home birth.

Learn what your insurance covers. Ask your friends and relatives which health care professionals they used, where they delivered, and what they liked or disliked. Here are the basic differences.

Hospitals

Most babies are born in hospitals. In a hospital you would get emergency care quickly, if necessary. You would not have to be moved to a hospital. (Most births do not require such care.)

Many hospitals:

- offer home-like birthing rooms
- allow your newborn baby to stay in your room
- allow birth partners to help you during labor and delivery

Think about what you would like. Ask about these services before you choose a hospital.

Birth center and home options

In some areas, parents can find ways to have less medical kind of care and a more home-like setting. You may be able to deliver at a birth center or at home. This can work well if you are healthy and expecting a normal birth. If a serious problem happened during labor, delivery, or afterward, you would be moved to a hospital right away.

Find out which doctors and hospital would be used if you needed to be moved in an emergency. Make sure that the hospital is close enough for safety.

Choosing a health care provider

You will want a professional you like and trust to give you care throughout your pregnancy and deliver your baby. This person will be very important to you during the next nine months.

Find out if your health plan gives you a choice of providers. Ask for a list of those who are included. The kinds of health care providers who give prenatal and birth care are:

Obstetrician-gynecologist: A doctor with special training in pregnancy, birth, and women's health. (Also called an "OB-GYN.")

Family physician: A doctor who gives primary care* to people of all ages. Do you already have a doctor who takes care of your family? He or she may care for you through your pregnancy. He could also provide care for your baby after birth. He would refer you to a specialist if you need one.

*Primary care: Basic health care for people of all ages

(If you use a naturopath for your regular care, make sure to find out if she is trained in prenatal care and when she would refer you to a specialist.)

Certified nurse-midwife* (CNM): Many CNMs work in hospitals and in birth centers. Some also deliver babies at home. In some states, midwives who are not nurses can be certified to give such care by taking a special test. If you want to use a midwife, make sure she is certified.

*Certified Nurse-midwife: A nurse who has had special training to deliver babies and who has passed a test.

I asked my friends about who they went to when they were pregnant. It was a big help to know if they would use them again.

Ask plenty of questions to find a health care provider you like. Look for a provider who:

- Is well trained and certified
- Listens to your birth choices (see Chapter 8)
- You can speak with (if English is not your first language)
- Has an office that you can get to easily
- Has an office with easy access if you have a disability or tty access if you are hard of hearing

You may want to meet two or three providers before choosing. They should be willing to meet with you at no charge.

The best health care provider for you

There are some important things about pregnancy and birth care to know before you choose your health care provider. So, before you meet with a health care provider, learn something about labor and delivery. This is a good time to read the first part of Chapter 6 and all of Chapter 10. Use the Glossary (in Chapter 17) to find the meanings of medical words you may not know.

Finding a doctor or nurse practitioner who understands your concerns will be important. Ask these key questions:

__ What training have you had in labor and delivery (if a family physician)?

__ Do you have other doctors or nurse-midwives who care for your patients when you are away? Will I have a chance to meet them?

__ Who can I call nights or weekends if I have a question or an emergency?

__ Do you encourage women to deliver in the position that they find best for them?

__ What medications do you prefer to use, if needed, to lessen pain during labor? Do you encourage methods other than drugs?

__ What methods do you usually use to avoid episiotomy*?

__ Do you like a woman to have a birth partner during labor and delivery?

__ In what situations do you recommend a cesarean section*? How frequently do you do non-emergency cesareans? (A rate of 15 percent is considered good.)

__ How do you advise a woman about vaginal delivery if she has already had a cesarean?

__ Do you encourage breastfeeding right after delivery?

Episiotomy: A cut made in the skin around the vagina to widen the opening and help the baby to be born.

*Cesarean section: Delivery of a baby through a cut through the woman's belly into the uterus.

If you have strong feelings about some of these things, be sure to discuss them before choosing a provider.

The most important question is to ask yourself: "Do I like this person? Will I be able to trust his or her* advice?"

During your pregnancy, you might you find are not happy with your doctor or nurse practitioner. Talk with the customer service office of your health plan. Find out what options you have to change providers.

*His or her (he or she) will be used to refer to a health care provider of either sex.

Prenatal checkups—what to expect

Your doctor or nurse practitioner will want to see you once a month until the last two months. During the last two months, you should have checkups more often. (You will find pages for keeping track of what happens at your checkups in Chapters 7, 8, and 9.)

Checkups allow the health care provider to keep track of how your baby is growing inside. He also will check your health. This is a good time for you to ask questions. It also is time for the provider to get to know you and how to help you. You should also have a chance to meet the other doctors or midwives who would care for you when your own provider is away.

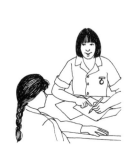

Your health care provider will check your weight, temperature, heart rate, blood pressure, breasts, and lungs. She will check the size of your uterus with a pelvic exam. A pelvic exam is done by reaching into your vagina with one hand and pressing on your belly with the other hand.

As your pregnancy goes along, she will use ultrasound to look at the baby's growth, the placenta, and the uterus. Usually, you and your partner will be able to see what shows on the ultrasound screen.

The pelvic exam is done while you lie on the table.

The doctor or nurse practitioner will also do certain laboratory tests with your blood and urine. These tests are to screen (check) for possible health problems. A test result that comes back "positive" means your provider would do other tests to find out more. If those tests also showed a problem, she would talk with you about what could be done to deal with it. If you do not understand, ask her to explain.

Talking with your provider

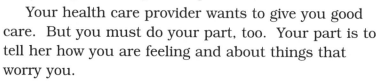

Your health care provider wants to give you good care. But you must do your part, too. Your part is to tell her how you are feeling and about things that worry you.

Write down concerns or questions as you think of them. (There are places to write questions on the checkup pages in Chapters 7, 8, and 9.) This will help you remember what to ask at your next checkup.

If you are not feeling well

Be sure to call your health care provider if you feel sick or your body seems different. Note the answers to these questions before you call:

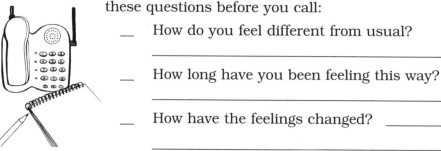

__ How do you feel different from usual?

_____

__ How long have you been feeling this way?

_____

__ How have the feelings changed? _____

_____

__ Do you have a fever? (Take your temperature and write it down before you call.) _____

Be sure to ask for more information if you don't understand the health care provider's advice.

Using medical services wisely

It is very important is to get prenatal care right away, even if you need help paying for it. Waiting until late in pregnancy can lead to unnecessary problems. Make sure your girl friends know they should get care early, too, if they think they might be pregnant.

Make appointments early so you can have a choice of time and day. If you have to cancel, call the office as soon as possible to let them know. Make another appointment to get the care you need.

Remember that it is always better to get a possible problem checked early, when it is easiest to treat. Waiting until it gets serious may be dangerous and costly.

Try to use the same doctor or clinic as much as possible. Use the hospital emergency department in true emergencies or at night when your regular clinic is not open. The emergency department is not set up to give regular care. The doctor or nurse there does not know your health history or that of your baby. Also, getting care there is very expensive.

Choosing your baby's doctor

Your baby will need a pediatrician,* family physician, or pediatric nurse practitioner* for health care. It is important to decide about this during pregnancy.

If you have a family doctor who provides you with on-going care, that professional can also care for your baby. If not, ask the provider who is caring for you during pregnancy to suggest a doctor for your baby. Ask your friends about their children's doctors. Check with your health plan for the providers on its list. Then meet with one or two doctors or nurse practitioners.

*Pediatrician: A doctor who has several years of special training in the health care of children.

*Pediatric Nurse Practitioner: A nurse with special training in children's care, who works with a family physician or pediatrician.

Some questions to ask before choosing:

- Does she have an office or clinic that is easy to get to? (You will need to take your baby there often for checkups.) Do the office hours fit your schedule?

- Is she friendly and easy to talk to, with time to answer questions? Does she have a nurse who can give you advice by phone when you need it?

- Is she easy to reach in an emergency? Who can you call when she is away?

- Do her concerns match yours? (Some parents have strong opinions about certain child health issues.)

Babies and children need to see their doctor or nurse practitioner regularly even when they are not sick. Usually babies have about six "well baby" checkups in their first year.

How will I pay for my baby's care?

If you have health insurance for your family, the plan will cover new babies. Be sure to call the plan soon after birth to tell them about your new child.

If you have no insurance, call your public health department or community clinic. These places can help you find care for yourself and your baby.

Chapter 6

Birth and Newborn Care

What you need to know now

Why is it important for you to think about birth and baby care now? Because there are some important things to learn and decide in advance. Also, it can take time to gather all the supplies and equipment you will need.

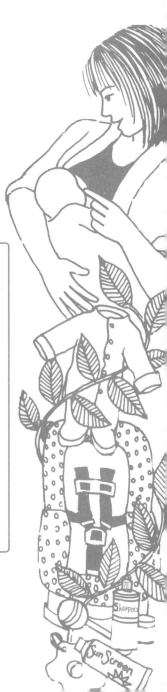

This chapter includes:

Birth choices, page 56

- Childbirth classes
- Concerns about birth choices
- Birth partners
- Maternity leave

Infant care, page 61

- Infant care classes
- Why breastfeeding is special
- Feeding with formula
- Things you will need for your new baby
- Choosing and installing a car seat

Preparing for childbirth

Why start so early?

It is not too soon to begin getting ready for the big event—your baby's birth. This is because it takes time to learn all you need to know. You also need to begin to learn about the choices that you may need to make about your care.

Do you worry about what labor and delivery will be like? This is normal. You may have heard stories that scare you. Or you may have had a delivery that was hard. The best way to cope with fear is to learn about what is happening to your body. No birth is without pain and hard work, but the more you know, the less painful your labor is likely to be.

How can I get ready?

Childbirth is a normal process. Women's bodies are made to the work of delivering a baby. It may seem strange but it is as natural as having sex. It is hard work, but your body will prepare for it. Most women feel proud and strong after they deliver a baby. The memory of pain quickly fades away.

The more you know, the more you can to make the birth go well. Read Chapter 10, which covers the basics. Sign up early for childbirth classes. Talk with friends about their experiences. Read other books for more details. Look on the Internet, too. (Books and Internet sites are listed in Chapter 17.) Find out all you can so you can make the best choices for you.

The most important things you can do to get ready for birth are:

- Learn about childbirth options. There are some choices that you may need to make that are not simple.

- Choose a birth partner. Having someone with you who knows something about the birth process can be very comforting during labor. This person (your baby's father or a close friend) would go to childbirth classes with you. He or she must be able to be with you when you go into labor.

- Go to a childbirth class. These are very important so you will know what happens during labor and delivery. Hospitals, health clinics, and childbirth groups give classes.

Childbirth class gives you confidence

A childbirth class is the best place to learn about labor and delivery. Knowing what will happen to your body will help it be easier and less painful. A class will give you the tools to be as comfortable as possible.

Even if you have given birth before, you may learn new things from a class. Every birth is different. Also, there may be new methods or new medications you do not know about.

There may be special classes in your area for people interested in specific kinds of natural childbirth, such as the Bradley or LaMaze method.

Classes usually last six or eight weeks. Sign up early to make sure you can get into a class before delivery. Some hospitals offer short refresher classes for people who have taken a class before. Ask about scholarships if you are not able to afford a class.

A childbirth class will teach you:

- How to prepare your body to help make labor easier
- Choices you can make about birth that your doctor or midwife will need to know ahead of time
- What happens during the stages of labor and delivery
- How to relax, breathe, and push to make the birth easier
- What kinds of medications can help if the pain is too much for you
- What would happen if you need a cesarean

Start learning now

Begin by reading Chapter 10. That covers the basics of birth, stage by stage. Talk with friends and your own mother about their experiences. However, remember that every woman and every birth is different.

Some women today feel frightened or disgusted by the idea of childbirth. You may hear that it is easiest to avoid it by taking a lot of painkilling drugs or having surgery. You may hear women say a cesarean section is easier.

Keep in mind the basic rule that heavy drugs or surgery should be used only when medically necessary. There are risks to using them. Drugs or cesarean delivery also take away many the positive feelings that come from having played an active part in the birth. Couples often feel closer after going through it together. Many husbands or partners admire their women for doing the hard work of childbirth.

Childbirth and pain

It is not possible to avoid all pain. Much of the problem with pain comes from not understanding what is happening. Pain that is normal is not scary. It goes away between contractions and almost as soon as your baby has been delivered. Even having a cesarean section is not pain free. There is a lot of pain for days or weeks when recovering from a c-section.

While there are various medications to reduce pain, there also are things you can do yourself. Walking around during early labor, using different positions later in labor, soaking in a warm bath, having a massage, breathing, and practicing relaxation methods all help. They help you feel better and help labor go more quickly.

Many medications have some side effects or can be used only at certain times.

Non-emergency cesarean delivery

Many babies are delivered by cesarean section today. Some of those surgeries are done for the health of the mother or baby, but most are not. Often they are done for minor problems that could be solved in other ways. Some women ask for a cesarean delivery, thinking it is easier and less painful.

Many doctors and nurse-midwives do not agree with surgery unless it is medically necessary. Research shows that mothers have many more complications from a cesarean section than from a normal delivery. Many major medical, nursing, and childbirth organizations say that the risks of surgery are higher than many women realize.

After surgery, a woman should expect to stay longer in the hospital, have less contact with her newborn baby, have severe pain for days or weeks, and take a long time to recover. Some other possible risks are:

- side effects of anesthesia
- infection, loss of blood
- difficulty starting breastfeeding
- injury to nearby organs
- less ability to get pregnant again
- more problems in future pregnancies

There are risks to the babies too. These include breathing problems at birth and a higher risk of asthma as children grow up.

Talk to your health care provider about how often he does cesarean sections. If he does it often, ask why. If you do not want surgery, you may need to find another doctor or hospital or use a nurse-midwife for your delivery.

Vaginal birth after cesarean

Many women who have had one cesarean may want to have a normal birth for the next delivery (called vaginal birth after cesarean or VBAC). This usually can be done safely, especially if your scar goes across your belly, not up and down. But not all doctors or hospitals allow it. Talk with your health care provider about the best method for you and your baby.

Who will help during birth?

You will probably want to have one or more birth partners. Nurses and doctors will come and go. A birth partner will be with you during the whole process.

During labor and delivery, your partner would help you by helping you remember and follow the breathing and relaxation methods you have learned. He or she would help you be as comfortable as possible.

"I was really glad my baby's father stayed with me all the way through delivery. He was a huge help. It meant a lot that he was there to know what I was going through."

Find someone who can go to classes with you and can take time out from work or away from family during delivery. You may want to ask two people, in case one cannot be with you during the whole time.

You may want to hire a doula. A doula is a woman trained and certified to help families during delivery. Care from this type of person can make the birth easier for both mom and baby. Most are in private practice (see Chapter 17).

Some people may think that birth would be very hard to watch. Your baby's father may not want to take part. Try to understand if he feels that way.

Maternity leave

Plan for maternity leave from your job. You will need some time to recover from birth. Ask for as much time off as possible. The first few months of parenthood can be exhausting. You and your baby also need time to get to know one another.

If you plan to breastfeed, talk with your employer about having a private place to pump your breasts after you go back to work. Using an electric pump will make it quick and easy to pump at work. Tell your employer that breastfeeding usually cuts down on a baby's illnesses. That will help you come to work regularly.

Learning about baby care

Learn as much as you can now. This is especially important because new moms and babies are usually sent home one or two days after delivery. You will not have time or energy for classes after your baby comes. There are many things to know more about, including breastfeeding, infant first aid and CPR,* home safety, and car seat use.

Four ways to learn:

- Read Chapters 11 to 15 for the basics. Read the rest of this chapter about the kinds of clothing, supplies, and equipment you will need before your baby is born.

- Go to new-parent classes at the hospital or birth center before your baby is born.

- Watch a video on infant care. Ask your health care provider for one.

- Spend time with other new mothers and babies.

*CPR: Cardio-pulmonary resuscitation, also called rescue breathing. CPR for infants is very different from CPR for adults. It is a life-saving method that must be learned before it is needed.

Breastfeeding your baby

It is important to learn and think about breastfeeding (also called nursing). If you are not sure you want to nurse your baby, you have time to find out more about it. You do not need to decide now. If you have decided, you might change your mind as your baby becomes more real.

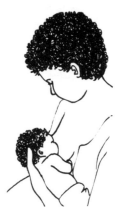

There is something very special about your newborn baby sucking at your breast. You are giving him the perfect food.

Touching your bare skin comforts him. It helps him makes the change from the womb to the outside world. It also can help you continue to feel close to the baby who has just left your body.

Why is breastfeeding the best choice?

- Human breast milk gives your baby exactly the right food for at least the first 6 months. It is the baby's most important food for at least the first year.

*Antibodies:
Cells made in the body to fight diseases. Breast milk provides a mother's antibodies to the baby.

- Breast milk gives your baby antibodies* that protect her from illness. She is likely to have fewer allergies, earaches, colds, diarrhea, and other problems. Formula cannot provide this protection.

- Breastfeeding helps you and your baby feel very close. This may be especially important when you go back to your job. Your baby can continue to drink breast milk when you are working.

- Breast milk costs nothing and is easy. There is no need to wash bottles, mix formula, or heat bottles.

- Breast milk is always clean, safe, the right temperature, and ready. You can feed your baby almost anywhere. You can breastfeed modestly in public.

"I like the idea of breastfeeding. Who wants to warm up a bottle in the middle of the night?"

- Night feedings are easy. There are no bottles to mix or warm up.

- Breastfeeding allows your baby to drink just as much as she needs. Breastfed babies are less likely to grow into overweight adults.

- It may take a little while for you and your baby to learn to breastfeed. However, it almost always works fine with a little practice and good advice.

- It is very rare for breasts to make too little milk if a baby breastfeeds 8 to 12 times per day and is given only breast milk. If a baby always seems hungry, he may not have latched on properly. You can learn how to get him to latch on well.

- The size of your breasts does not matter for breastfeeding. Their size is not related to the milk glands inside. If your breasts are usually small, you may enjoy having them be larger for a while.

For more about breastfeeding, see Chapter 12.

Starting with breast milk makes sense

Your milk in the first weeks is especially healthy. This is a good reason to try breastfeeding. You probably will like it. Even breastfeeding for a few weeks or months is better for your baby than not doing it at all.

Many, many mothers are able to breastfeed easily. For the few who have problems at first, there usually are easy answers. You will be able to get help and advice from people who have experience breastfeeding.

If you do not breast feed at the beginning, your breasts stop making milk. After that, you cannot go back to breastfeeding. You can switch from breast to formula later if you want to.

Bottle-feeding with breast milk

Babies can learn to take breast milk from a bottle after breastfeeding is going well. If you are going back to work, you can pump your breast milk and store it. Dad or other caregivers can feed your milk to your baby when you cannot be there.

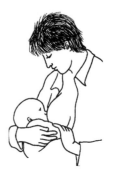

Health benefits to moms who breast feed

You will find that breastfeeding helps you lose the weight you gained during pregnancy. Breastfeeding now also helps protect you from some kinds of cancer and osteoporosis (bone thinning) later in life.

If you are not sure

If you are not sure you want to breastfeed, think about why. Have other people tried to talk you out of doing it? Maybe you heard other young mothers or your own mother talk about difficulties with breastfeeding. Maybe you do not know other young women who have nursed their babies.

Remember that every baby is different. Breastfeeding will also be different for each mother. Your mother may have used formula, but we know much more today about the health benefits of breast milk. Moms who have stopped breastfeeding early may not have had good advice getting started.

"My best friend told me, 'When I am nursing, I know I'm doing something no one else can do for my baby. And I feel very feminine and beautiful, even if my hair's dirty and I didn't get much sleep last night.'"

Take time to think about all the good things about breastfeeding for both your baby and yourself. Ask friends and co-workers about their experiences. Seek out people who have breastfed for more than a month or two. Find out from them how nursing really is.

Breastfeeding does not have to tie you down. By the time you are ready to go out without your baby, you can give him a bottle of breastmilk or formula.

This decision should be yours. If you have never done it, you have no way of knowing just how it will be for you. You CAN do it if you want to.

Feeding with formula

Formula is artificial breast milk. It is made to be as much like breast milk as possible. It is the only kind of milk to give your baby if you decide not to breastfeed. Here are some things to think about.

Breastfeeding vs. Formula Feeding

• Breast milk has antibodies and many, many nutrients	• Formula has the main nutrients but no antibodies. Babies may have more colds, ear infections, and diarrhea.
• Breast milk is free	• Formula is expensive.
• Breast milk is always ready for baby	• Formula must be mixed, stored, and warmed properly.
• Breasts need no special clean up after nursing	• Bottles and nipples must be washed with soap and hot water each day.

Things your baby will need

Now is a good time to start thinking about getting clothes, a car seat, and other baby things. It takes time to collect everything a baby needs.

Friends and thrift shops are good sources of baby clothes. If you are looking for bargains, beware of second-hand car seats and cribs. They may have serious safety problems. For more about safety, see Chapter 14.

Clothes

☐ **Warm sleepers with legs, Tee shirts with snaps under the crotch, socks, a warm hat.** Start with the 3- to 6-month size. Most babies outgrow the smallest size very quickly. If your baby is born early and is small, he could use newborn clothes at first.

☐ **Diapers:** Which kind is best? There are benefits and problems with disposable and cloth diapers. A diaper service or disposable diapers can be easy to use but usually cost more than washing your own. Some moms wash their own most of the time and use disposables when they take their babies out.

Equipment

☐ **A car safety seat*** that fits a new baby. Use it on every ride, starting with the trip home from the hospital. This is the law in every state and protects your baby from the biggest danger to his life. (Find more about choosing a car seat later in this chapter.)

*Car safety seat: A special kind of seat for use in motor vehicles. Also called a "car seat" or a "child restraint."

☐ **A crib or cradle** for your baby to sleep in, with a firm mattress that fits snugly, plastic mattress cover, and several sheets.

At first, you could use a small cradle or basket. As your baby gets bigger, you will need a large crib with high sides. The sides must have narrow spaces between the slats, 2³/₈ inches or less. (This is about the width of a soda can.) Beware of older cribs with wider spaces that could catch a baby's head. Some have other safety problems, too, like posts and cut-outs in the head and footboards.

Supplies

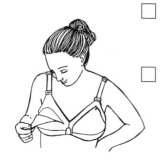

☐ **Nursing bras for you.** These open in front to make breastfeeding easier. Buy these somewhat bigger than you need while you are pregnant.

☐ **Medicines that babies may need:** including "non-aspirin" liquid pain reliever (such as Tylenol) for fever. (Aspirin can be harmful to babies and young children.) Zinc oxide ointment is helpful for diaper rash. Ask your doctor or nurse about other medicines that you might need to have on hand.

☐ **Thermometer:** Have a digital thermometer to use if your baby has a fever. Do not use a glass thermometer. A glass one has mercury in it, which is very poisonous if the glass breaks.*

*If you have an old glass thermometer, do not throw it in the trash. Take it to a hazardous waste collection site.

☐ **Bottles, nipples, and formula:** You will only need a few bottles for use with breast milk. For formula feeding, you will need at least 8 bottles.

☐ **Thin, small receiving blankets** for swaddling your baby.

Other useful things

☐ **A nursing pillow:** a curved foam pillow that fits around your body on your lap. Your baby can lie on it while nursing.

☐ **A baby tub:** A shallow plastic tub with a sloping back or a foam cushion will help keep your wet, soapy baby safe and make bath time easier.

☐ **A rocking chair:** Rocking in your arms in a chair makes many babies feel happy and peaceful. A baby who is fussy also may like being in a swing for short periods.

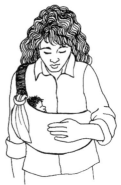

☐ **A reclining infant seat:** An infant seat that rocks or bounces can be calming but should be used only for short periods. Use it only when an adult is with the baby. (When a baby is awake, she needs time to lie on her tummy and to be held. When she is sleeping, she should be lying flat on her back.)

☐ **A cloth baby carrier:** Use a sling or front pack for holding your baby when you do chores or go walking or shopping. A sling-type carrier (see picture) may be easier to put on than a carrier with more buckles and adjustments.

☐ **A pacifier:** Sucking can calm a fussy baby, but not all babies or parents need pacifiers. Your clean finger or baby's own fingers are a natural pacifier. Pacifiers during sleep have been shown to help prevent SIDS. If your baby has colic, a pacifier can be very helpful.

Choose a pacifier made in one piece. This is safest because the nipple cannot come off and be swallowed. Be sure not to tie the pacifier around your baby's neck. The string could strangle him.

☐ **Baby toys:** Small rattles and bells make sounds that babies like. Soft and washable toys are good choices. They should not have small hard parts (such as plastic eyes) that your baby could chew or pull off. These could choke a baby. Avoid long strings that could get wrapped around her neck.

☐ **A mobile:** Babies like to look at dangling toys with parts that swing or turn. Hang one over your baby's bed or changing table. Get one with bold black and white or brightly colored shapes that are easy for your baby to see. Choose one with shapes that show from below. Hang it high out of reach.

☐ **Books and pamphlets:** Collect information on baby care from your clinic, doctor's office, or bookstore. Look on the Internet for more. See Chapter 17 for books and web sites that are helpful and that you can trust.

Second-hand things

Used clothing and some other baby things can be a real bargain at re-sale shops. Little babies do not wear out their clothes and toys. You often can get very good quality things at resale shops that are only slightly used.

Beware of some used equipment. Second-hand car seats, cribs, playpens, and some toys often have serious safety problems. It may be better to buy these things.

Car seats:

Newer car seats have many improvements. Older ones may have a number of problems. You need to know:

- **Has the car seat been used in a crash?** A car seat should not be used after a crash that is more than a fender-bender. This is because it may have hidden damage. If you cannot find out, do not use it.

- **Does it have its instructions and parts?** It is important to follow the instructions because not all car seats work the same way. You can get new instructions or replacement parts from the manufacturer (check their websites).

- **How old is it?** Because of advances in design, most manufacturers recommend not using car seats more than six years old. Car seats older than 10 years must be thrown away. (Take them apart first, so they cannot be taken out of the trash and re-used.)

- **Has the car seat been recalled?** Many recalls are for serious safety hazards. To find out, call the manufacturer with the model number and date of manufacture. If a used seat does not have a sticker with the date and number, you cannot check it.

Cribs:

Many older cribs have unsafe designs and may have been recalled. There is a standard for safe cribs, but even some new cribs do not meet the standard. Use a crib with narrow spaces between the slats so a baby's head cannot get trapped between them. It also should not have posts or knobs that stick up in the corners. Stay away from cribs with holes or cut-outs that your baby could get his neck stuck in.

Playpens:

Do not use a playpen with sides that fold down. These can trap a baby's neck.

Gates:

Safe gates have two parts that adjust by sliding sideward. Beware of old gates that have diamond-shaped holes and fold like an accordion. They can strangle a baby.

For product recall information, see Chapter 17.

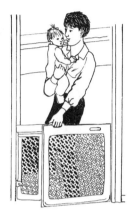

Choosing a car seat

Your hospital will expect you to take your baby home in a car seat. A car can be the most dangerous place for a baby or older child. Car safety seats do a very good job of protecting children in crashes.

Which is the best car seat?

There is not one "best" car seat for everyone. The best one for your new baby is:

- Made to be used rear-facing for an infant
- Able to fit and be buckled into your vehicle tightly
- Easy to use correctly, so you will use it on every trip

A more expensive seat is not always safer. All must pass the same tough safety tests. The fit of the car seat in your car and for your child are most important.

This is one product that is best to buy new (see Second-hand things, page 68). If you cannot afford one, ask your hospital, clinic, or auto insurance company if they offer low-cost car seats. If not, start saving now.

Two kinds of car seats for babies:

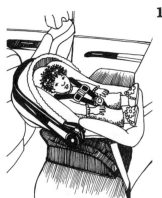

An infant-only car seat fits newborns well and is convenient to carry.

1. Small car seat for infants only, weighing less than 22 pounds (up to about 8 to 10 months of age). An infant-only seat (see picture, left) can be very useful for a newborn. (Never use a household infant seat, which is not built to protect in a crash.) This kind:

   • Is lightweight, easy to carry from car to home

   • May have a base that can be left installed in the car.

   • Costs less, but will be outgrown soon

   • May fit in a stroller base

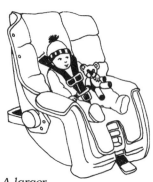

A larger convertible car seat with a harness fits children from birth up to 40 pounds.

2. Convertible car seat: This kind fits babies and children up to 40 pounds and about age 3 to 6. It can be used facing the rear for a baby and facing forward when the child is older. A convertible car seat has:

   • A harness (see lower picture) or a padded shield and shoulder straps. Pick a seat with a harness, not a shield, for a newborn babies.

   • Higher rear-facing weight limits (30 to 35 pounds) than an infant-only car seat. This allows a baby to ride facing the rear up to 18 months or 2 years of age.

Learn how to use the car seat

Get the car seat early. Practice putting a baby doll into the seat and adjusting the harness. Practice installing the car seat into the car facing the rear.

Turn to Chapter 14 for details about using the car seat correctly. Follow the car seat and vehicle instructions. Many car seats are not used properly.

"I am shocked when I see a family in the car with the kids riding loose in the back seat. Don't they know how dangerous that is?"

Not every car seat fits well in every car. If the one you have does not fit tightly in the car or you have questions, have your seat checked before the baby comes. Find a trained Child Passenger Safety Technician in your area (see Chapter 17).

Chapter 7

First Trimester:
Months 1, 2, and 3

Weeks 1 through 13

Your whole pregnancy will last about nine months. It can be divided into three parts, called "trimesters." This chapter will guide you through the first trimester. The next two chapters will cover the other two trimesters. Chapter 10 deals with labor and delivery.

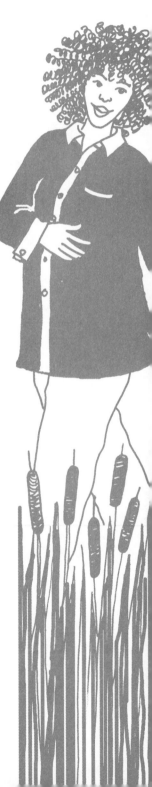

This chapter includes:

Months 1 and 2, page 73

- First checkups
- Your baby in your body
- Taking care of yourself in the early months

Month 3, page 82

- Third-month care and checkup
- Eating well and gaining weight
- Warning signs to know
- Common concerns: Miscarriage, Birth defects

How long does pregnancy last?

Doctors and nurse-midwives often talk about the number of weeks of pregnancy. This is because your unborn baby grows and changes so much during each week. There will be about 40 weeks from your last period until your baby's birth.

This is how the weeks and months are divided up:

1st trimester = months 1–3 = weeks 1–13

2nd trimester = months 4–6 = weeks 14–27

3rd trimester = months 7–9 = weeks 28–40

Most women feel quite different during each trimester. During the first, you and your body will be getting used to pregnancy. In the second trimester, you will probably feel more comfortable and content. In the third, you may be less comfortable. You will be looking ahead to delivery and parenthood.

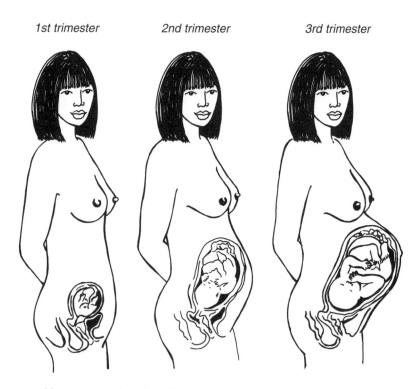

1st trimester   *2nd trimester*   *3rd trimester*

How your body changes as your baby grows

How is my baby growing?

Month 1 (1 to 5 weeks after your last period)

Your unborn baby is too small to see at the very beginning. After 4 to 5 weeks, he* will grow to be almost as big as a peanut.

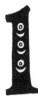

- His brain and spinal cord, lungs, and heart are forming.

- His head has little spots where his eyes will be.

Remember, this book will use "he" or "she" for any baby, male or female.

Look back at the life-sized pictures of growth in the uterus (Chapter 3, page 20). See the baby's amazing growth in the first few months.

Your second month (6 to 9 weeks)

Now the tiny unborn baby is beginning to look like a person. He has tiny eyes, ears, and a mouth. He will grow to about one inch (25 millimeters) long, about the size of a walnut.

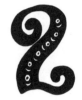

- He now has the beginnings of all the organs and systems that he will have at birth.

- Arms and legs are forming, with tiny fingers and toes.

- His heart is beating, pumping blood around his body.

"It is hard to believe that he already has fingers and toes. I hardly feel pregnant yet!"

- His brain is growing very fast, so his head is much larger than his body.

Changes you will notice

- Your skin may be drier than usual.

- Your face may break out. There may be changes in color across your nose and cheeks.

- You may start to get a dark line down the middle of your belly.

- Your nipples will get darker and your breasts will swell.

- Your breasts and belly will get larger and may get ribbon-like stretch marks.

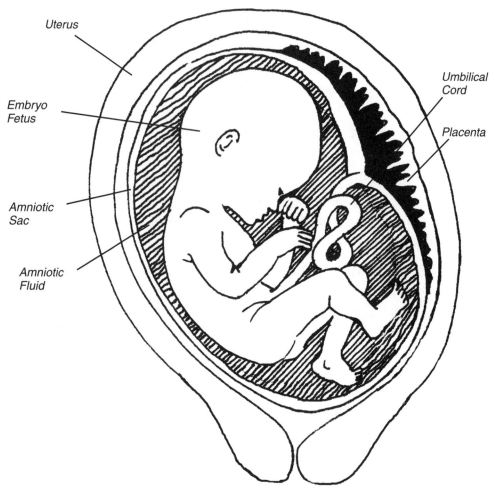

Uterus

Embryo
Fetus

Amniotic
Sac

Amniotic
Fluid

Umbilical
Cord

Placenta

Here is where your unborn baby grows

*Words in bold
are shown in
the picture.*

Your baby in your body

Your unborn baby lives in your **uterus** (womb). He
is called an **embryo** during the first 8 weeks. After
that time, he is a called a **fetus.** He curls up in the
amniotic sac (bag of waters) filled with **amniotic fluid.**

The **umbilical cord** and the **placenta** connect your
baby's body to your body. The placenta is attached to
the wall of your uterus. The blood in the placenta and
cord carry food, oxygen, and other things to your
baby's body. It also carries some things that could
harm your baby, like alcohol and nicotine.

Your first prenatal visit

Your doctor or nurse-midwife will give you a complete examination. This is what usually happens at this visit. The doctor or nurse will:

- Ask questions about your health history and habits. Tell her as much as you can. Things you may not like to talk about could make a difference in your care. The same could be true for things that do not seem important. The more your provider knows, the better care she can give you.

- Ask about the health of your parents and relatives. Some health conditions of other family members could affect your health and your pregnancy.

- Measure your height, weight, temperature, heart rate, blood pressure, breasts, and lungs.

- Do a pelvic exam to find out the size and position of your uterus.

- Ask you to give blood, urine, and other samples to test for conditions like chlamydia, hepatitis B, and HIV. Your provider needs to know about any problems as soon as possible.

- Give you a prescription for prenatal vitamins.

HIV-AIDS test: Important for every pregnant woman

A blood test for HIV, the virus that causes AIDS, is important because:

- Many women do not know they are infected with HIV.

- If a woman has HIV, she should get special care right away. Her doctor can help make sure she and her unborn baby get the best care.

- There are drugs that can reduce the chance that an unborn baby will get HIV from his mother.

Your health care provider should talk with you about the test before and after you take it. If you have HIV or AIDS, there are things you can do to cope with this disease.

All about me (notes before my first checkup)

I am ___ years old. My birthday is _____.

(month, day, year)

I am _____ inches tall and weighed _____ pounds before I got pregnant.

My last menstrual period started on _____.

(date)

- Health problems I have (illnesses, surgeries, etc.):

  _____
  _____
  _____
  _____

- Health problems in my family (husband or partner, my other children, my parents, brothers, sisters):

  _____
  _____
  _____
  _____

- Medicines, herbs, and supplements I use:

  _____
  _____
  _____
  _____

- **Questions I have about being pregnant:**

  _____
  _____
  _____
  _____
  _____
  _____
  _____

All of the things you have listed are important to talk about with your doctor or nurse-midwife.

Record of your first prenatal visit

Date _____ (usually 4 to 8 weeks after your last period).

I am about ___ weeks pregnant.

I weigh ____ pounds today.

My blood pressure is _____.

Tests I had today: _____

_____

_____

_____

_____

_____

My doctor or nurse-midwife's name* is

_____

Office phone: _____

Emergency phone: _____

*Put this name and both phone numbers in the front of this book. Also post them by your phone, so they will be easy to find.

Things I learned today

1. My baby's "due date" is _____

_____

2. _____

_____

_____

3. _____

_____

_____

My next checkup will be on

The _____ of _____, at ___:___.
    (date)   (month)   (time)

Signs of an Emergency

Know the warning signs of a problem during pregnancy. Read about them on page 88 later in this chapter. Call your health care provider if you think you might have any of them.

How can I take care of myself?

Some of your baby's most important growth happens in the first two months. Remember and practice the healthy habits in Chapters 2 and 3.

- Go to your checkups and learn about pregnancy.

- Keep your body free of tobacco, alcohol, and drugs. Stay away from places where others are smoking.

- Have a dental checkup and have any gum disease treated.

- Eat the healthy foods that your baby needs.

- Get plenty of exercise and rest.

- Wear your safety belt on every car ride.

- Take time to relax.

- Make sure to protect yourself from STDs if you have more than one sex partner.

- Don't use medicines you have around the house. First ask your health care provider if they are safe. There are ways to treat many common health problems, such as colds, without taking medicines.

How can I keep from feeling so tired?

In the first few months, you may feel very tired. Learn to say "no" if you would rather rest than go out with friends. Your energy will return in the second trimester.

What if my stomach feels upset?

In the early months, you often may feel like throwing up. You may even vomit daily. This is called "morning sickness" but it can happen at any time of day. It usually stops after the first few months of pregnancy. Here are some ways you can cope with it.

- Eat smaller meals every two or three hours. Do not wait until you feel really hungry. Eat a small snack before going to bed.

- Eat some plain crackers before getting out of bed in the morning or when you feel sick. Keep them beside your bed.

- Sip a little plain soda water.

- Eat the foods that you feel hungry for. You may like foods that you didn't like before. Do not worry if the food you can keep in your stomach is not the most nutritious. You can eat better foods after the morning sickness is over.

- Stay away from greasy or spicy foods if they make you feel sick.

- Drink water or weak tea with a little sugar if you have been vomiting. This gives your body back the liquid it has lost.

- Take your vitamins with food. They can upset your stomach if it is empty.

Call your doctor or nurse-midwife between checkups if you are vomiting every day.

Breaking habits

You know that smoking, drinking alcohol, or taking drugs can harm your baby. Are you finding it hard to quit using any of them?

There are ways to break these powerful addictions. Talk with your health care provider about ways to stop. Your health insurance plan or health care provider may offer programs to help people stop smoking. Your doctor or nurse-midwife also can help you get drug or alcohol counseling.

Healthy teeth and gums

Gum infections can affect your baby's health by increasing the risk of preterm labor. Have a dental checkup early in pregnancy. Keep your teeth and gums healthy by flossing and brushing daily.

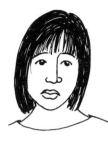

Moods are normal

Why do I feel happy one minute and sad the next?

In the first three months, you are likely to have strong feelings of sadness and happiness. This may surprise you, but it is normal. Hormones in your body change during pregnancy. This may cause these feelings. Most women's moods settle down after the first trimester.

You may have fears or worries about delivery or your baby's health. These thoughts are normal, too. Learning more will probably make you less afraid.

- Are you worried about your baby's health? Learn more about the real risks and what you can do about many of them.

- Are you worried about what birth will be like? A childbirth class will help answer your questions. You can also read books and pamphlets. (See the book list in the back of this book.)

- Are you worried about being a good parent? Start learning now about how to care for your baby. You may be able to practice by caring for a friend's baby.

Things to do to help you feel better:

- Learn to cook some new and healthy recipes.

- Take a walk every day. Do it with a friend so you can talk together while you walk.

- Try learning something new, like knitting. You could make a hat for your baby.

- Do something nice for someone, like babysitting for a friend or visiting an elderly neighbor.

- Have a girls' night out with your friends to see a funny movie.

- Talk about your feelings or have a good cry when you feel blue.

Talking about feelings can help

Telling someone who cares about you often helps you feel better! This might be your baby's father, your mother, your sister, or your best friend. Choose people who will really listen to you. They will be more helpful than people who try to tell you what to do.

Who would you want to tell if you feel upset?

1. _____

2. _____

3. _____

How do you feel now?

_____
_____
_____
_____
_____

What worries do you have?

_____
_____
_____
_____
_____

What makes you feel happy now?

_____
_____
_____
_____
_____

Should I tell my doctor or nurse-midwife?

Yes, these people want to know about your moods and worries. Be sure to call if you feel like this for more than two weeks:

- Very sad or empty

- Unable to sleep or sleeping all day long

- No appetite or eating all the time

Learning more about pregnancy and baby care

You can find information about birth and infant care in many places. Look in Chapter 17 and search on the Internet. Ask for a list of local resources at your clinic. Check at your local library, the health department, or WIC office. Look in the community pages in the front of your phone book.

The local hospital and community college often have classes on pregnancy and baby care. You may have to sign up ahead of time.

How do you know the things you learn are correct? Know the source of information you hear or read. Is the sponsor (person, article author, or web site) professionally qualified? Check any new information with your doctor or nurse-midwife before you decide to change what you are doing.

Your third month (10 to 13 weeks)

How is my body changing?

- You are starting to gain weight. By the end of this month, you probably will have gained 2 to 5 pounds in all. To be comfortable, you will need some larger clothes soon.

- By the end of this month, you may be able to feel your uterus. Press your fingers into your belly just above your pubic bone. You will feel something round and hard like an orange. That is the top of your uterus.

- Your breasts will probably feel very heavy and may hurt. This is normal. Make sure you wear a bra that fits well.

- You may get constipated more often than before you got pregnant. Eat plenty of fruit, bran, and prunes to prevent this. Ask your doctor before taking any medication for constipation.

How is my baby growing?

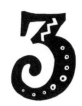

- By the end of this month, your baby will be about 4 inches long.
- Your baby will weigh about one-half ounce and is now called a fetus instead of an embryo.
- His heart is beating very fast. It is loud enough for your doctor or nurse-midwife to hear.
- Fingers and toes are completely formed.
- Arms and legs can move now. Your baby is still so small that you cannot feel the kicks.

What can I do to stay healthy?

- Eat plenty of vegetables, fruits, and whole grain breads.
- Take your prenatal vitamin pill daily.
- Drink plenty of water instead of sweet soft drinks or diet sodas. For a healthy drink, try fruit juice mixed with soda water.
- To get some exercise, walk as much as possible instead of driving. Take the stairs instead of the elevator to go up one or two flights.
- Stay out of smoky rooms. Ask friends who smoke not to do it inside your home or car.

Questions to ask at my next checkup

- What can I do if I am constipated?
- Why do I feel so happy one day and so sad the next?
- Am I gaining enough weight?
- How will I know if I am having twins?
- I am having trouble quitting smoking. What will make quitting easier?

Other questions I have:

1. _____

2. _____

3. _____

My three-month checkup

After the first visit, most checkups will probably be simple and short. Your weight, blood pressure, and the size of your uterus will be measured. You will be asked to give a urine sample. Your provider will check your baby's heartbeat. (Soon you will be able to hear it, too.) Be sure to ask any questions you have.

Ultrasound: A tool to see the fetus inside the uterus. Pictures show on a screen.

At some visits, you may have tests, such as ultrasound,* to see how the baby is growing. Ultrasound will show how the parts of the body are developing and possibly the sex of the fetus. (Tell your health care provider if you want to know the sex of the baby before birth.) You should be able to see your baby on the ultrasound screen.

On this date, _____, I had my three-month appointment.

I am ____ weeks pregnant.

I weigh ____ pounds now.

I have gained ____ pounds since my last checkup.

My blood pressure is _____.

Things I learned today

1. _____
   _____
   _____

2. _____
   _____
   _____

3. _____
   _____
   _____

My next checkup will be on

The _____ of _____, at ____:____.

    (date)   *(month)*   *(time)*

Do I have to "eat for two"?

You do not need to eat twice as much as before you got pregnant. Most pregnant women need to eat only a little more than usual. The important thing is to eat healthy foods so you and your unborn baby get the best nutrition possible.

Will I gain too much weight?

It is healthy to gain weight while you are pregnant. Look at the chart on the next page. You can see that many parts of your body get heavier as the months go by. Your body changes to grow your baby and get ready for birth. Most women lose that weight after their babies are born.

Gaining too little weight can cause preterm labor. The baby may be small at birth, which also can cause health problems. However, gaining too much weight is not healthy either. If you are very heavy when you get pregnant, talk with your doctor or nurse-midwife.

This is not the time to diet! If you limit the healthy foods you eat, your baby's food is limited, too. Also, diet pills are drugs that could be especially harmful to your unborn baby.

Are you afraid to gain weight? Do you diet often or make yourself vomit to stay thin? These habits could harm you and your baby's health. You can get help by talking about this problem with your doctor or nurse-midwife.

How much weight gain is healthy?

How much is best for you depends on your weight before you got pregnant. Talk with your doctor or nurse-midwife about how much weight gain is healthy for you. Limit your food only if your health care provider asks you to.

A healthy gain for women of normal weight would be between 20–34 pounds. If you are very thin, you should gain more. If you are heavier than average, you should gain less. If you are overweight, your doctor may want you to gain as little as 10 pounds. If you are pregnant with twins, you can expect to gain more (40 or more pounds).

You are not gaining only the weight of the baby. Many parts of your body will get heavier as pregnancy goes along. The box below shows how much weight parts of your body will gain.

Weight Gain During Pregnancy

Parts of the body	Weight at delivery (average)
Your baby	6 to 9 pounds
Uterus and Amniotic fluid—where your baby grows	4 pounds
Placenta—connects mother and baby	2 pounds
Breasts—prepare to make milk	1 to 4 pounds
Extra blood in your body	4 to 5 pounds
Fat—stored energy for labor and breastfeeding	4 to 6 pounds
Total	**21 to 30 pounds**

Teenage weight issues

If you are a teenager, remember that your body is also still growing. It is very important to eat enough for your own growth and the baby. Your doctor or nurse-midwife will help you understand how much weight gain is right for your age.

Limit the junk food that is so easy to buy or fix. It may spoil your appetite for the nutritious foods you and your baby need.

Keeping up your healthy habits

How are you doing? You probably have been making some big changes in your life and activities. Many pregnant women must work hard to change how they eat, sleep, or exercise.

It is hard to break old habits. These might be eating too many potato chips or candy bars or much more serious habits like smoking, drinking, taking drugs, or not exercising. Have any of these things been hard for you?

What have been the hardest things to change?

_____

_____

What has been the easiest to change?

_____

_____

Who has helped you the most in making changes?

_____

_____

What healthy habits are you still working on?

_____

_____

_____

_____

_____

_____

Would you like help?

If you need help starting healthy habits, ask for it. Your baby's father, your friends, and your family will want to help. They do not always know what you need unless you tell them.

Signs of an emergency

Know how to reach your doctor or nurse-midwife. Call right away—day or night—if any of these things happen:

- Bleeding from your vagina
- Painful cramps in your belly or back
- Strong headaches, dizziness, vision problems
- Fever or chills
- Swelling of your hands, feet, or face
- Painful reddish area on one leg or pain when walking
- Very rapid weight gain
- Lessening of activity of the fetus (later in pregnancy this could mean a problem with the fetus—see Chapter 9)

Common concerns

Having twins?

Tests can be done to check the number of embryos early in pregnancy. If you are having a "multiple" pregnancy, there are some extra risks. Your health care provider will talk with you about the special care you will need. With good care and healthy habits, you are very likely to have healthy babies.

You may:

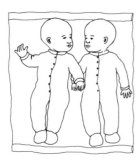

- Gain more weight than with a single baby
- Need more rest (lying on your left side is best)
- Go to checkups more often later in pregnancy
- Have preterm labor (see Chapter 8)
- Need a cesarean section

Could I lose my unborn baby?

Many pregnancies end naturally during the first three months. Sometimes it happens in the fourth or fifth month. This is called a miscarriage or spontaneous abortion.

An early miscarriage usually happens when there is something seriously wrong with the embryo or fetus. A problem with the mother's health (an infection, the condition of the uterus or placenta, or a serious injury) also could cause miscarriage. You may never know why it happened. Miscarriages are not caused by anything a pregnant woman normally does, such as working hard or having sex.

The signs that a miscarriage is starting are bleeding, cramps, or backache. It is important to talk with your health care provider if you start having any of these signs. Most miscarriages cannot be stopped.

When miscarriage happens in the first few weeks of pregnancy, it may seem like a late, heavy menstrual period. If it happens later, there usually is heavy bleeding and very painful cramps.

After a miscarriage, your health care provider should check your uterus. It is important to make sure that no parts of the embryo (or fetus) or placenta are still inside.

Expectant parents often feel very sad for weeks or months afterward. If you have lost your unborn child, these feelings are very natural. Others may not understand your sadness, especially if the miscarriage happened early. It usually helps to talk with others who also have had miscarriages or read about pregnancy loss.

After your uterus heals, you have a very good chance of getting pregnant again and having a normal pregnancy. Talk with your doctor or nurse-midwife about any problems in your body that might have led to the miscarriage. Ask how soon to try again and whether you need to prepare in any way. Meanwhile, be sure to keep your body healthy (see Chapter 1).

Could my baby have a birth defect?

A small number of babies are born with birth defects (health problems that begin before or during birth). Some defects are serious, but others are not. Some can be found before delivery but others cannot.

Does any member of your family have a birth defect? If so, it is a good idea to talk with a genetics counselor as early as possible.

Causes of birth defects

- A health problem of the mother. (Example: If a mother has German measles in early pregnancy, her baby might have hearing, heart, and eye problems.)

- Something that gets into the mother's body and harms the fetus. (Example: Alcohol can cause serious defects in the brain and body.)

- A problem that happens during birth. (Example, too little oxygen for the baby during delivery could cause brain damage.)

- A "genetic" defect that is caused by problems in parents' genes. (Example: Sickle-cell anemia is a genetic disease that can be passed down from parent to child.)

- Unknown causes.

*Amniocentesis: A test of the fluid inside the bag of waters, showing certain things about your unborn baby's health.

Some defects show up in ultrasound, special blood tests, or amniocentesis.* If these tests show a possible problem, other tests would be done. Your health care provider would talk with you and your partner about what to do and may refer you to a specialist.

Ask your health care provider or genetics counselor which tests would be helpful to you. Learn about the tests so you can decide if you want them. If your unborn baby has a defect, it is often helpful to know early. You and your health care providers can prepare to take the best care of your baby.

Check your health insurance policy or benefits office to find out what genetic services are covered.

Chapter 8

Second Trimester: Months 4, 5, and 6

Weeks 14 to 27

During the second trimester, most women feel better than in the first three months. Your body is getting used to having a new life growing inside. You are getting used to the idea of being a mom.

This trimester is a time when your body will begin to change shape. Exercise becomes more and more important.

By six months, you will be planning for your baby's birth. Look back at Chapter 6. During this time, you can start learning about baby care. This is a good time to begin collecting the clothing and other things your baby will need.

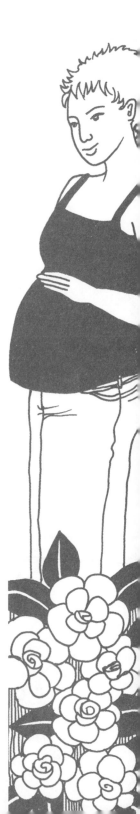

This chapter includes:

Month 4, page 92

- Exercises (pelvic tilt, kegel, stretches)
- Sex during pregnancy

Month 5, page 98

- Preventing constipation
- Signs of preterm labor, page 101

Month 6, page 103

As your body starts to change shape, your baby's father may become more interested in your pregnancy. Share this book with him. Invite him to come with you to your checkups.

Remember: Every prenatal checkup is important. If you miss a visit, call right away and set another date.

Your fourth month (14–18 weeks)

How is my body changing?

- You are starting to gain weight more quickly, and will gain about 1 pound each week from now on.
- Your breasts are still large, but may be less tender.
- You may not need to urinate as often as during the past months.
- If you had morning sickness, you may start to enjoy eating again.
- You may have more energy again.

How is my baby growing?

- At the end of this month, your unborn baby will be up to 7 inches long. She will weigh about three-quarters of a pound.
- Soft hair, called "lanugo," grows on her body. Eyebrows and eyelashes appear.
- She will be able to suck and swallow.
- She will move enough for you to feel tiny kicks. They may feel like flutters or rumblings of gas.

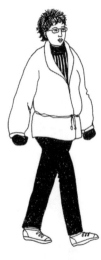

What can I do to stay healthy?

- Go for your regular checkups.
- Stay away from cigarettes, smoky places, alcohol, or any drugs.
- Take a half-hour walk every day or two. For the best workout when you walk, go fast and swing your arms. Wear flat, cushioned sport shoes.
- Drink eight glasses of water every day.

- Have healthy foods on your kitchen shelf to have when you feel like a snack.
- Take only the vitamins or medicines that your doctor or nurse-midwife has told you to take. Take the right number each day.

Questions to ask at my next checkup

- Is my blood pressure normal?
- Can I keep playing sports and exercising?
- I have not felt my baby move yet. How do I know she is okay?
- If I have had a cesarean section before, must I have one this time?

Other questions I have:

1. _____

   _____

2. _____

   _____

My four-month checkup

On this date, _____, I had my four-month appointment.

I am ____ weeks pregnant.

I weigh ____ pounds now.

I have gained ____ pounds since my last checkup.

I have gained ____ pounds since I got pregnant.

My blood pressure is _____.

Things I learned today

1. _____

   _____

2. _____

   _____

My next checkup will be on

The _____ of _____, at ___:___.
   (date)   (month)   (time)

Delicious and healthy snacks

- **Fresh fruits**—orange, apple, peach, or papaya with non-fat yogurt on top
- **Dried fruits**—raisins, apricots, or prunes mixed with roasted pumpkin seeds, peanuts, or almonds
- **Raw vegetables**—carrots, tomatoes, or broccoli dipped in a little salad dressing
- **Popcorn**—without oil

What to do about heartburn?

A painful feeling in the middle of your chest (heartburn) after eating is common in pregnancy. It is caused by acid backing up into the tube from your mouth to your stomach. Try these tips:

- Eat smaller meals more often.
- Chew your food well.
- Stop eating any foods that make your heartburn worse.
- Eat several hours before going to sleep and lie with your head and chest raised about six inches.
- Wear clothes that are loose around your middle.

If these things don't work, ask your provider what medicines you can take safely to help you feel better.

Swollen legs

Do your legs and your feet swell when you stand up for a long time? Try:

- Wearing support hose,
- Putting up your feet when you are sitting,
- Moving around often,
- Standing with one foot up on a low stool or box,
- Wearing flat shoes that have plenty of room for your toes,
- Eating fewer salty foods and drinking fewer diet sodas.

Shape up for pregnancy

These exercises help your body stay strong through your whole life.

1. "Kegel squeeze" helps birth muscles

This exercise (named for a Doctor Kegel) strengthens the muscles around the opening of your vagina. Those muscles hold up your growing uterus. This exercise also helps hold your vagina and bladder in place as you get older.

An easy way to learn this exercise is while you are urinating on the toilet. Here's how:

- Squeeze your vaginal muscles to stop or slow the flow of urine. Try **not** to tighten your stomach muscles or buttocks.

- Hold tight while you count 1–2–3–4–5.

- Relax, and then squeeze again. (After you know how this exercise feels, don't do it on the toilet.)

You can do the Kegel squeeze anywhere. Try it standing at the kitchen sink or waiting for the bus. Practice until you can do it 25 times, three or four times a day.

2. "Pelvic tilt" lessens low back pain

Strengthen the stomach muscles (see pictures) to help prevent low back pain.

- Rest on hands and knees with your back straight. Breathe in and relax your back.

- Breathe out, tighten your stomach muscles and pull your buttocks under you. Your back will arch. Count to five. Then breathe in again and relax your stomach.

- Now try it standing up. Tighten your stomach and pull your buttocks under. Repeat this as often as possible each day.

Pelvic Tilt:
Your pelvis tilts up when you arch your back and pull in your buttocks. It tilts down when you relax.

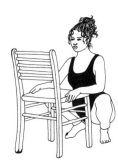

Squat holding onto a chair for balance.

3. Squatting and sitting cross-legged

These two ways of sitting loosen your hips and the joints of your pelvic bones. They also stretch your inner thighs. **Both can help with back pain now. They also will help when you are pushing your baby out.**

- To squat, start with feet apart. Hold onto a chair so you do not fall. Squat down, keeping your heels on the floor, if possible. (Don't try this if you have knee problems.)

- Sit cross-legged on the floor. Spread your knees wide apart and cross your ankles. For more stretch, put the soles of your feet together.

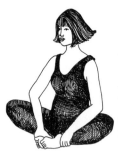

For more stretch while sitting on the floor, put your feet together.

4. Standing straight and tall

Standing with your back very straight can lessen low back pain. It also helps you look slim and feel good about yourself. To see how this looks, do it in front of a long mirror.

- Stand sideways to the mirror with bare feet. Pull your chin in and your head up.

- Bring your shoulders down and back. Pull your belly in and your buttocks under. This is like doing the Pelvic Tilt.

See how your belly and buttocks look smaller. Feel how your muscles work together. Practice standing and walking this way. Soon it will become a habit.

Learning to lift with your legs

It will help you greatly if you can always squat to lift heavy things. This saves your back from a lot of stress during pregnancy. It also will be important when you have a baby. When he starts to play on the floor, you will often need to lift him up.

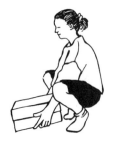

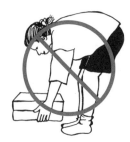

The right way to lift.   *The wrong way to lift.*

Keeping the loving feeling during pregnancy

You both may find that your enjoyment of sex is changing. As your belly grows larger, sex may become less enjoyable. However, some women find it more exciting. Your partner may have different sexual feelings, too.

You can try new ways to enjoy sex. Tell your partner what positions feel best now. Try lying on one side, with your partner behind you. Many women find that position the easiest as their belly gets bigger.

There are many ways to enjoy being together. Talk about the kinds of touches that feel good to you. At times, just being close and holding each other can be enough. This is an important time to talk about what you are thinking and feeling. Remember that you will feel sexier after you heal from giving birth.

Having sex will not harm your baby if your pregnancy is normal. It does not make labor start. Sometimes, however, the doctor or midwife may tell you not to have sex. Sex could be harmful to the baby's health if you are having bleeding or after your waters have broken.

If any blood or water comes from your vagina, stop having sex. Call your doctor or nurse-midwife right away.

It is still important to protect yourself from sexually transmitted diseases. Both partners must get treatment if either one has an STD. This is essential to an unborn baby's health.

Painful breasts

As your breasts grow larger and heavier, they may hurt. A firm bra that fits well will keep them as comfortable as possible. You may want to wear a bra for sleeping, too.

Your fifth month (19 to 23 weeks)

How is my body changing?

- You will now be gaining about 3 to 4 pounds each month.

- The top of your uterus may be up to your belly button.

- The skin on your face may get light or dark patches. A dark line may run down the middle of your belly. These changes will disappear after pregnancy.

- You will probably have plenty of energy and feel very well this month.

How is my baby growing?

- At the end of this month, your unborn baby will be up to 12 inches long. He is more than half as long as a newborn baby.

- He will weigh almost one and one-half pounds. This is about as much as a large (24-ounce) loaf of bread.

- His skin is very wrinkly. A thick white coating called "vernix" covers it.

- He moves enough now for you to feel his kicks easily. He does not move all the time.

- Hair is starting to grow on his head.

What can I do to stay healthy?

- Go for your regular checkups.

- Continue to stay away from cigarettes, alcohol, drugs, or second-hand smoke.

- Walk in different places (the mall or the park) so you don't get bored. Invite a friend along.

- Be sure to drink eight glasses of liquids each day.

- Eat plenty of healthy foods, like vegetables, beans, whole wheat breads, and yogurt. Save sweets for special treats.

- Take prenatal vitamins every day.

Questions to ask

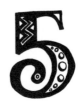

- Is my baby growing well?
- How could my job be harmful to my baby?
- Is there any chance I could be having twins?
- Where can I find a good childbirth class?
- How long should I keep on working?
- Is my blood pressure normal?
- What can I do about varicose veins?

Other questions I have:

1. _____
   _____

2. _____
   _____

My five-month checkup

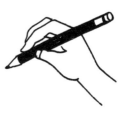

On this date, _____, I had my five-month appointment.

I am ____ weeks pregnant.

I weigh ____ pounds now.

I have gained ____ pounds since my last checkup.

My blood pressure is _____.

Things I learned today

1. _____
   _____

2. _____
   _____

3. _____
   _____

My next checkup will be on

The _____ of _____, at ____:____.
   (date)   (month)   (time)

Braxton Hicks contractions

You will start to feel your uterus getting hard for few moments and then relaxing. These are Braxton Hicks contractions. These are painless and can happen any time—close together or a long time apart. These contractions happen more in the later months of pregnancy. This is nothing to worry about. Your uterus is preparing for labor.

When labor begins too soon

Sometimes real labor starts before 37 weeks. This is called preterm labor. Often preterm labor can be stopped to give the baby more time to grow inside.

Every additional day a baby spends in the uterus helps him be more ready for life outside. A baby born too early may have health problems. Some babies born as early as 24 weeks can survive, but only with lots of special care.

It is important to know the signs of preterm labor. These signs do not always mean preterm labor has started. However, it is best to call your health care provider right away if you think you might need special care.

Take action right away. Your doctor or nurse-midwife may want you to come to the office or the hospital right away. Or she may ask you to take a rest for an hour first, lying on your left side. She may want you to drink two or three glasses of water or juice. Sometimes these things are enough to stop the contractions.

Some women are more likely to have preterm labor than others. Be sure to talk with your doctor or nurse-midwife right away if you have:

- Twins or a multiple pregnancy
- Unusual stress
- Gum disease
- Vaginal diseases (chlamydia, bacterial vaginosis)

Warning signs of preterm labor

Call your provider right away if you have any of these signs:

- Bleeding or pink or brown liquid coming from your vagina
- Loss of the mucus plug or clear water leaking from the vagina
- Contractions every 10 minutes or less, or cramps like those during your period
- Low backache that may be steady or come and go
- Heavy feeling in your pelvis and vaginal area, like the baby might fall out
- Unusual tightness or hardness of your belly
- A general feeling that something is wrong

What can I do about constipation?

It is easier to keep your bowel movements soft than to fix constipation. Here are some ways to make sure you do not get constipated.

- Exercise every day.
- Drink 8 to 10 tall glasses of liquids every day; half should be water.
- Eat foods with plenty of fiber, such as fresh fruits and vegetables, brown rice, and whole grain bread or cereal.
- Eat a few dried prunes before bed every night.

If you get constipated often, take more prunes or drink warm prune juice. Ask your doctor or nurse-midwife if you need a stool softener.

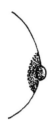

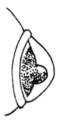

Nipple shell

Nipple shapes for nursing

Some women's nipples stick out naturally more than others do. All will work for breastfeeding. If yours look flat, try squeezing them around the edge of the areola (dark area). If they do not stick out more when you squeeze, they are inverted. Talk with your health care provider about your nipples if you are concerned.

They may stick out more as pregnancy goes on. If they do not, you could try using breast shells (lower picture). Wear them over your nipples inside your bra. The shell presses around the base of the nipple, pushing the nipple out. Do this for a few hours a day during the last few months of pregnancy. Nipple shells can be found where breastfeeding supplies are sold.

After birth, a breastfeeding consultant can help if your baby does not latch on easily. Your baby needs to suck on the areola (the dark part around the nipple) not only on the nipple. Once your baby is sucking well, your nipples should stay out.

Especially for father

Getting ready for baby's birth

Show this page to your baby's father, if he hasn't read the whole book!

Dad, you are essential to your unborn baby's life, birth, and growth. Here are some things to do as you wait for birth.

- Feel your unborn baby move by putting your hand on your partner's tummy.

- Talk to your baby about things you will do with him after birth.

- Go to checkups with your partner.

- Go to childbirth classes and practice the breathing exercises with her between classes.

- Help pick out the baby's car seat. Learn how to use it correctly. (See Chapters 6 and 14.) Read the directions and practice securing it in the car. This is a very important way to keep your baby safe.

- Talk about names you like for your baby.

- If you think you do not want to see the birth, say so. You could help during labor and leave the room when the delivery starts. You can be a good father without seeing your baby born.

- Having sex will not harm your unborn baby, if your partner's pregnancy is going well. However, she may not enjoy having sex in the weeks before and after birth. Talk with her about what feels good to her. Find out what positions are comfortable for her. Ask her what kind of touching she would like.

  Do not try to have sex if your partner is bleeding, the bag of waters has broken, or she is having preterm labor. Call the doctor or nurse-midwife instead.

If you feel left out by your partner at this time, tell her. She may be thinking about her unborn baby most of the time. Talking with each other about how you are feeling is a healthy habit.

Take time together to do things that will be harder after your baby is born. Visit friends. Take a few days off for a vacation. Go to the movies. Get plenty of sleep!

Your sixth month (24 to 27 weeks)
How is my body changing?

- The top of your uterus is now above your belly button.

- You may feel contractions as the muscle of your uterus tightens and then relaxes. These are normal contractions called "Braxton-Hicks." They mean your uterus is getting ready for labor.

- You will probably have a good appetite now.

- You may get stretch marks on your belly and breasts. Your belly may itch as your skin stretches. (Lotion may help stop the itching.) Your belly button may pop out.

- Your legs may get cramps at night and your ankles may swell.

How is my baby growing?

- At the end of this month, your baby will be up to 14 inches long. That is about the length of your arm from elbow to fingertips. She lies curled up, her knees against her chest.

- Your baby will weigh about 2 pounds. This is as much as a half-gallon of milk.

- Her eyes are almost completely developed. She can open and close her eyelids.

- She can hiccup and suck her thumb.

- You will feel her kicking.

What can I do to stay healthy?

- Continue eating many kinds of healthy food. Fish, chicken, lentils, beans, fruits, and vegetables are important for your baby's growth.

- Keep away from people who are smoking. Put off drinking beer or wine until after birth and breast-feeding are finished.

- Sign up for a childbirth class.

- Join a prenatal exercise group if you have a hard time exercising by yourself.

- Take some time to have fun with friends before your baby comes. You might plan a picnic in the park, a movie, or a quiet dinner together.

- Remember to buckle your seat belt whenever you drive or ride with others. Push the lap belt down under your belly and pull it tight. Keep the shoulder belt snug across your upper body.

Questions to ask at my next checkup

- Is there any reason not to try breastfeeding?
- Am I likely to go into preterm labor?
- Why do I feel my baby move often on some days and less on others?
- How do I know if I am getting enough exercise?
- Are my nipples ready for breastfeeding?

Other questions I have:

1. _____

   _____

2. _____

   _____

My six-month checkup

On this date, _____, I had my six-month appointment.

I am ____ weeks pregnant.

I weigh ____ pounds.

I have gained ____ pounds since my last checkup.

My blood pressure is _____.

Things I learned today

1. _____

   _____

2. _____

   _____

3. _____

   _____

My next checkup will be on

The _____ of _____, at ____:____.
　　(date)　　　　(month)　　　　　(time)

Diabetes during pregnancy

Some women get diabetes while they are pregnant (called gestational diabetes). This can cause serious problems for both mother and baby. Most health care providers give a test for this condition at about 26 weeks. If you have it, you can learn to control it. Gestational diabetes usually goes away after birth.

For mothers who are Rh negative

Your health care provider will tell you if your blood is Rh negative. This means that your blood does not have a substance called the Rh (Rhesus) factor. You would need special care during pregnancy if your baby has the Rh factor. If you need it, your doctor would give you a special substance (Rhogam) at about 28 weeks. Ask if you need this treatment.

Talking to your baby

"The kids gave our unborn baby a nickname. We all ended up calling him 'Bobby' instead of 'baby.'

Soon your unborn baby will be able to hear sounds from outside the uterus. He may learn the sound of your voice. Talk to him about how you are getting ready for his birth.

If you have other children, tell them about the baby inside your body. Let them feel your belly when your baby is moving. Invite them to talk to the unborn baby.

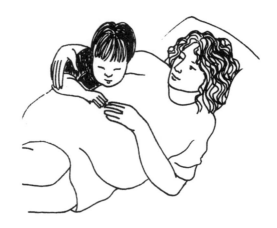

Chapter 9

Third Trimester: Months 7, 8, and 9

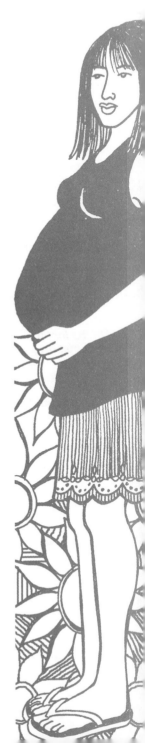

28 to 40 weeks

Your third trimester (months 7, 8, and 9) is starting. Your pregnancy is almost over. You have done a lot to help your baby be healthy. Are you eager to get started being a parent?

Your body has been preparing for birth for months. If you have not done so, read Chapter 10 and take a childbirth class. Get busy learning about infant care, too. You will not have time with a new baby in the house. Your community probably has infant care classes.

Most important: Check page 101 (Chapter 8) to be sure you know the signs of preterm labor. You may get tired of pregnancy, but your baby needs to

---

This chapter includes:

- How to get comfortable

Month 7, page 109

- Warning signs—high blood pressure, page 111

Month 8, page 112

- Counting baby's kicks
- Making a birth plan

Month 9, page 122

stay safely inside your uterus until at least 38 weeks. Call your health care provider right away if you think labor might be starting.

How your growing baby affects your body

Many organs are pushed out of place as your baby grows. These are normal ways your body will feel different when the uterus gets larger:

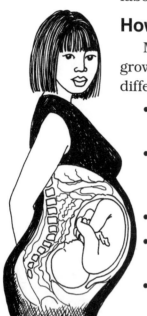

- When your baby presses up against your **lungs**, you may feel short of breath.

- Your stomach and intestines may have a harder time digesting the food you eat. Large meals may make you uncomfortable.

- Your bowel movements may be harder to push out.

- Your bladder, which holds urine, will be squeezed. You may need to urinate more often.

- Your breasts will swell and ache, as they get ready to make milk after birth.

Ways to get more comfortable

In the last three months, the growing baby pushes against your lungs, stomach, and intestines.

- Wear a bra in bed if your breasts ache and feel heavy.

- Lie on your side with pillows supporting your belly, between your knees, and behind your back. Try different pillow positions to see what feels good to you.

- Sit in a straight chair. To get up, move to the edge of the seat and lean forward. Then use your leg muscles to get up.

- Try not to sit too long without moving. While sitting, point your toes and rotate your feet to help blood flow. Sit with your feet raised.

- If you have to stand for long periods, wear comfortable shoes with low heels.

- Practice standing straight with your chin in, your tummy muscles firm, and your buttocks tucked under. Try putting one foot up on a low stool while you stand.

- Wait a while after eating before you lie down.
- Eat a number of small meals instead of three large ones.
- Sit cross-legged on the floor to relax your lower back.
- Continue to do the exercises in Chapter 8.

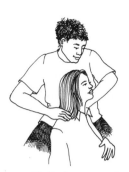

"It feels so good to have my partner rub my shoulders."

Your seventh month (28 to 32 weeks)

How is my body changing?

- You could gain another 4 pounds this month.
- Your bulging belly may make you feel awkward. Your hip joints are getting looser and may ache. This also can make you feel clumsy. You may feel dizzy when you stand up suddenly.
- You may feel kicks against your ribs. You may see your belly bulge as your baby moves.
- You may feel hot and may sweat more than usual. Wear light, loose clothing to stay cool.
- Colostrum may leak from your breasts.

How is my baby growing?

- At the end of this month, your baby will be up to 16 inches long. She will weigh about 4 pounds.
- Her body is well formed. She would have a good chance of surviving if she were born now.
- You may feel her hiccup. She can even suck her thumb!

Watch for signs of preterm labor. This is especially important if you are having twins or multiples.

Include your children in your pregnancy

As delivery gets closer, make sure you pay attention to your other children. Talk about the baby who is coming. Read some books together about new babies. Give them a doll so they will have their own baby. All

"I realized that my baby would be born in November, so I decided to get my children's Christmas gifts early in the fall. It was great to have all that done before my baby was born."

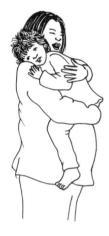

Make sure your older children know you will have plenty of love for all of them.

these things will help make this big change seem more natural. Let them know that you will still love them after the baby is born.

If you plan to move them into other bedrooms, do it a few months before the baby is born. You may want to get a supply of larger clothes for them so you will not have to go out shopping too often with a new baby.

What can I do to stay healthy?

- Go to your prenatal checkups.
- Go to your childbirth classes. Encourage your birth partner to go with you. Between classes, practice the exercises that you learn.
- Drink at least 8 glasses of water every day.
- Do gentle exercises like walking every day.
- Be sure to rest every day with your feet up.

Questions to ask at my next checkup

- How long should I plan to keep working?
- Am I likely to go into labor early (preterm labor)?
- Do I have inverted nipples?
- I eat lots of vegetables, fruit, and grains but still get constipated. What else can I do?
- When should I start counting how often my baby moves?
- If you are expecting twins: Is there anything special I should know to prevent preterm labor?

Other questions I have:

1. _____

   _____

2. _____

   _____

My seven-month checkup

Today, _____, I had my seven-month appointment.

I am ____ weeks pregnant.

I weigh ____ pounds.

I have gained ____ pounds since my last checkup.

My blood pressure is _____ (see below).

Things I learned today

1. _____
   _____

2. _____
   _____

My next checkup will be on

The _____ of _____, at ____:____.
   (date)   (month)   (time)

Watch out for high blood pressure

High blood pressure during pregnancy (called preeclampsia, toxemia, or PIH) can become dangerous to you and your baby. It is most likely to happen with a first pregnancy. If your blood pressure is high, you will need to take special care of yourself to prevent more serious problems.

These signs may mean that PIH is getting worse:

- sudden weight gain (more than a pound in a day)
- headache
- swelling of hands and face
- blurred vision or spots before your eyes
- nausea and vomiting

You may need emergency care. Call your doctor or nurse-midwife right away!

Your eighth month (33 to 36 weeks)

How is my body changing?

- You will gain about 4 more pounds this month.

- The top of the uterus is reaching your ribs. You may have trouble breathing when your baby pushes against your lungs.

- Your hands and feet may swell.

- Your body may feel very warm. Light, loose clothes will help.

- You may need to urinate often as your baby presses on your bladder. You also will have less control of when you urinate or leak urine when you sneeze.

How is my baby growing?

- Your baby will be about 18 inches long and weigh about 5 pounds.

- She can open her eyes and see light.

- She may move less than last month. There is less room to turn over inside the uterus now.

- Your baby will settle into one position in the uterus. She may be head down or buttocks (bottom) down.

- Your belly will bulge when the baby pushes on it. Can you feel her head, feet, and elbows?

What can I do to stay healthy?

- Go to 2 checkups this month.

- Go to childbirth classes.

- Keep up your healthy habits. Stay away from alcohol, drugs, cigarettes, and smoky places.

- Take time to take a walk every day, even if you move more slowly now. Practice the exercises in Chapter 8 and those you learn in your childbirth class.

- Be sure you are eating plenty of foods rich in calcium—dry beans, milk, tofu, peanuts, dark green vegetables.
- Put your feet up whenever you sit down.
- Choose your baby's doctor or clinic. Be sure to tell your own doctor about your decision.

Questions to ask at my next checkup

- Is my baby growing well?
- Can my partner and I still have sex and what positions are best at this time?
- Is my baby lying head down or head up?
- How is my blood pressure?
- Is it healthy to keep exercising as I get closer to delivery?
- Should I register at the hospital or birth center before I go into labor?

Other questions I have:

1. _____

   _____

2. _____

   _____

Decide about circumcision

If your baby is a boy, do you want him circumcised? This is a choice for you and your baby's father to make together. Circumcision is usually done soon after birth. There is no clear medical need to do it, but you may have religious or personal reasons.

Uncircumcised penis

Time to choose a baby doctor

Now is the time to choose the doctor or nurse practitioner for your baby if you have not yet done so. Look back at Chapter 5 for tips on this important decision.

Circumcised penis

First 8-Month Checkup

On this date, _____, I had my first eight-month appointment.

I am ____ weeks pregnant.

I weigh ____ pounds.

I have gained ____ pounds since my last checkup.

My blood pressure is _____.

My baby's position: _____.

Things I learned today

1. _____
   _____

2. _____
   _____

My doctor or nurse-midwife wants me to call when I have these signs of labor:

1. _____

2. _____

3. _____

4. _____

My next checkup will be on

The _____ of _____, at ____:____.
    (date)   (month)   (time)

Count baby's kicks

Pay special attention to how often your baby moves. Babies have quiet and active times each day. But babies usually move at least 10 times in 1 to 2 hours. Count your baby's kicks and punches daily.

An easy way is to keep track of how long it takes for your baby to move ten times in a row. You could do this sitting quietly with your feet up. Note the start time and make a mark for each movement on a piece of paper. When you reach ten, note the ending time and the length of time. It might take 10 minutes or an hour.

If your baby isn't moving, she may be asleep. Try waking her with a loud noise. Try counting again in an hour or two.

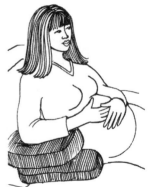

Call your health care provider right away if your baby has slowed down a lot or stopped moving completely for 10 to 12 hours. The doctor may want to do tests to see why she is less active.

Avoiding an episiotomy

An episiotomy (ep-easy-oto-me) is a cut made in the perineum to make more space for the baby to come out. An episiotomy is not always necessary. It can be painful after birth.

The perineum needs time to stretch wide open as the baby's head pushes against it. If the delivery is slow, no cut may be needed. Sometimes the perineum tears, but this is often much smaller than an episiotomy.

Ways to protect your perineum:

- Massage your perineum during the few weeks before delivery. (See directions, page 118)

- Make sure your health care provider knows you want to avoid being cut. She can help stretch the perineum during delivery.

- Follow what the nurse-midwife or doctor says when pushing, so the baby does not come out too fast.

Test for strep infection

One kind of infection that a mother might pass to her baby is Group B Strep (GBS). This can be very serious for a newborn. Mother and baby must be treated at birth. Some health care providers test all pregnant women at 35 to 37 weeks. Ask your doctor or nurse-midwife if you need the GBS test.

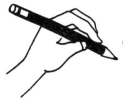

My second eighth-month checkup

On this date, _____, I had my second eight-month appointment.

I am ____ weeks pregnant.

I weigh ____ pounds now.

I have gained ____ pounds since my last checkup.

I have gained ____ pounds since I got pregnant.

My blood pressure is _____.

Things I learned today

1. _____

_____

2. _____

_____

3. _____

_____

My next checkup will be on

The _____ of _____, at ___:___.
   (date)   (month)   (time)

How your body changes

Braxton Hicks contractions that you have been feeling for several months help the uterus get ready for labor. The uterus is one big muscle that is very strong by the time labor starts. If you have already given birth at least once, you will probably feel them more.

The joints in your pelvis are becoming loose. This allows the pelvic bones to spread apart to make more room for the baby to go between them. As this happens, the baby in the uterus moves down and the bulge of your belly drops.

Your breasts will start leaking colostrum. Wash your nipples with clear water. There's no need to use soap. It could dry the skin of your nipples.

Your baby is starting to move down into the birth canal. This is often called "dropping" or "lightening." You will notice that your belly seems lower and you can breathe easier. You may find you need to urinate more often as your baby presses on your bladder.

Your cervix begins to thin and open (see pictures below). You will not feel this happening. These changes will speed up when you go into active labor. The thick mucus that has plugged your cervix may come out with a small amount of blood (called "bloody show.").

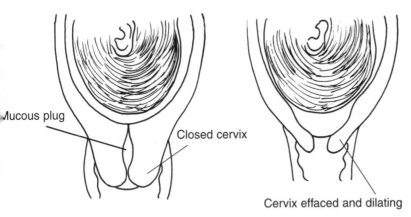

Mucous plug

Closed cervix

Cervix effaced and dilating

How your cervix opens

Effacement is the thinning of the neck of the cervix. Dilation is the opening of the hole. Both things happen as the baby's body presses down on the cervix.

When you visit the doctor or nurse-midwife in the last few weeks of pregnancy, she will check:

- How far down the uterus has moved into the pelvis
- How much the cervix has thinned (effaced)
- How wide the mouth of the cervix has opened (dilated)

Your health care provider also will feel your baby's position. Most babies turn so their heads are down before delivery. If the baby's position is bottom down (breech) or sideward, your doctor or nurse-midwife may try to turn him. If labor starts with the baby in the breech position, a cesarean birth will usually be done for your baby's safety.

While you wait

You can do many things to get your body ready for labor. Continuing the exercises and stretches from Chapter 8 as long as they are comfortable.

When you feel your uterus getting tight (Braxton-Hicks contractions) and hard, you can practice relaxing. Try the breathing methods from your childbirth classes and the other ways of dealing with the discomfort of labor and delivery. Try the positions that can help during the different stages. These are all ways to help the contractions do their work and reduce your stress.

Practice tightening and relaxing your pelvic floor (perineum) using the Kegel Squeeze. Relax your perineum by letting it bulge out. You also can stretch it by massaging it during the last six weeks to reduce the likelihood of tearing.

How to massage your perineum

Wash your hands. Stand with one foot up on a chair. Squirt a little vegetable oil or K-Y Jelly on your thumb. (If you have long nails, cut this one short.) Reach inside your vagina with your thumb and relax your muscles. Move your thumb side to side, pressing out and down toward your anus. Stretch your perineum for about three minutes several times per day.

How to be comfortable now

When you are standing and sitting, it is very helpful not to slouch. Standing straight, pulling in your belly, helps prevent back pain.

It is hard to get comfortable lying down when your belly is large. Lying on your back may make you feel dizzy. Lying on your left side works best. Put one pillow under your belly and another between your knees.

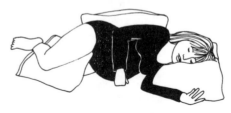

Talk to your baby

Remember, your baby can hear the sounds you make. Does she ever move when she hears sounds? Talk to her about how you are getting ready to be her parent. Tell her about her family.

Making a Birth Plan

It is a good idea to write out a plan before birth. This will be very helpful if you will have a hospital delivery, where the caregivers may not know you personally.

There are different ways to do most of the things that happen during a normal birth. It is good to think about them before you are in labor. At that time, it would be hard to think clearly.

Make your plan after learning as much as you can about birth. Be sure to talk it over with your health care provider. Talk about your options with your doctor or nurse-midwife. Get her thoughts about the best care and why she advises certain choices. If you feel strongly that you want as little medical treatment as possible—or if you want as little pain as possible—your provider needs to know.

Ask your childbirth teacher if she has a form you can use. If not, use the form on the next page. Have your plan put into your medical record and keep a copy to bring to the hospital.

Birth does not always go according to plan, of course. Every birth is different. You can always change your mind during labor. Your condition may change. If the doctor or nurse-midwife has an important reason to change the plan, make sure she explains it to you.

A birth plan:

- Who will be your birth partner or partners?

  _____

- Do you want to be able to move around during
  labor? _____

- Drugs: Do you want to use pain medication? If
  so, what kinds?_____

  How will you decide to take them? _____

- What positions do you want to use during labor?
  (such as standing, sitting, or squatting)

  _____

- Do you want to try to avoid having an episiotomy
  and prefer other methods to avoid tearing the
  skin around your vagina? _____

- Who will cut the cord? _____

- Do you want to breastfeed your baby right away?

  _____

  Do you want the nurses to give her no formula
  or water? _____

- Do you want your baby to stay in your room all
  the time? _____

- In case of a cesarean birth, would you like to be
  able to watch or have the doctor explain what is
  happening? _____

  Does your birth partner want to be there? _____

- Will a baby boy be circumcised? _____

  Do you want medication to be used to reduce the
  baby's pain? _____

  Do you and your partner want to be present?

  _____

  Will it be a religious ceremony? _____

- Other things you want the doctor and nurses to
  know:

  _____

  _____

Last steps to get ready

You are probably very tired of waiting, but you will go into labor soon. It can seem very hard to wait.

Check the signs of labor

Look ahead to Chapter 10 to review what will happen during labor and delivery. Learn the signs of labor so you will be prepared.

Register ahead of time at the hospital

Call the hospital or birth center and ask how to register early. That would make it easier for you to be admitted when you arrive in labor.

Pack your bag for the hospital stay

Have everything ready ahead of time. (See list, Chapter 10.)

Plan how to get to the hospital

Decide who will take you to the hospital or birth center. Make sure the person taking you knows how to get there. If you have never been there, go once to learn the way. Have a second person ready to drive you in case the first driver cannot do it. If you live far from the hospital, you may want to go there earlier than usual.

"We lived an hour's drive from the hospital. When labor started, we drove to a friend's house that was close to the hospital. Then we didn't worry about delivering on the highway."

Plan for help after birth

Ask some friends or family members to help around the house for a few weeks after delivery. Some families hire a doula to help at home and offer support for newborn care.

Your children and birth

Let your older children know that you will be going to give birth soon. Tell them what arrangements you have made for their care while you are away. If you are having a home birth, it is still very important to have someone to care for them.

Your ninth month (36 to 40 weeks)

How is my body changing?

- You will probably gain about 4 more pounds in this month.

- Sometime this month, the baby will move down into your pelvis. Breathing and eating may be more comfortable after this happens, but you may need to urinate more often. You also may get constipated more easily.

- You may feel very tired. This is normal. Give yourself time to rest.

"Just before my baby was born, I cleaned all the kitchen cabinets completely. I was amazed that I had the energy for it."

- Just before labor begins, you may feel new energy to do things around the house. This is called "nesting." This is a good time to pack your bag with things to take to the hospital or birth center. Try not to get tired out. You will need your strength for birth.

How is my baby growing?

- Your baby is gaining fat to help her keep her body temperature up. Her lungs are getting ready to breathe air. Most babies are about 20 inches long at birth. Most weigh about 7 pounds.

- All the parts of her body are well formed now. She could be born any time.

- Her fingernails are getting longer.

- She has grown to fill the uterus and has little room to move. She may seem quieter.

Things to have ready at home:

- Some cooked meals in the freezer

- Menstrual pads (not tampons)

- Diapers and other baby supplies

- Mild laundry soap for baby's clothes

What can I do to stay healthy?

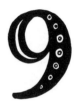

- Be sure to eat prunes, whole wheat bread, fresh fruits, and vegetables.

- Do your relaxation and breathing exercises.

- Get plenty of rest with your feet up.

- Make your birth plan. Talk it over with your doctor or nurse-midwife.

- Go for your checkup each week.

Questions to ask at my next checkup

- How will I know if my contractions are real labor? When should I call you?

- What positions (sitting, squatting, or lying down) do you think work best during labor?

- If I need pain medication, what kinds would you advise? What side effects would they have for my baby and me?

- Who can I turn to for help with breastfeeding?

- Do I need a Group B Strep test?

Other questions I have:

1. _____
   _____

2. _____
   _____

3. _____
   _____

Use the last page of this chapter to write things you want to remember about this important time.

My first ninth-month checkup

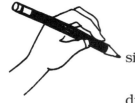

On this date, _____, I had my first nine-month appointment.

I weigh ____ pounds now.

I have gained ____ pounds since my last checkup.

My baby has dropped? Yes ___   No ___

I am ___ percent effaced and ___ centimeters dilated. (This may not be measured at every checkup this month.)

My baby's position is head down ___ or bottom down ___.

Things I learned today

1. _____

_____

2. _____

_____

My next checkup will be on

The _____ of _____, at ___:___.

     (date)   (month)   (time)

My second ninth-month checkup

Date _____

I weigh ____ pounds and have gained ___ pounds since I got pregnant.

I am ___ percent effaced and ___ centimeters dilated (if measured).

Things I learned today

1. _____

2. _____

My next checkup will be on

The _____ of _____, at ___:___.

     (date)   (month)   (time)

My third ninth-month checkup

Date _____

I weigh ____ pounds now.

I am ___ percent effaced and ___ centimeters dilated (if measured).

Things I learned today

1. _____

2. _____

My next checkup will be on

The _____ of _____, at ____:____.
     (date)   (month)   (time)

My fourth ninth-month checkup

Date _____

I weigh ____ pounds now.

I am ___ percent effaced and ___ centimeters dilated (if measured).

Things I learned today

1. _____

2. _____

How I am feeling now

_____

_____

You can keep a record of what happened during labor and delivery at the end of Chapter 10.

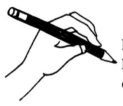

The big day is almost here!

Whether your pregnancy has been easy or not, you know it will end soon. You will soon have a new child to love. You have already started to be a parent by taking care of your unborn baby.

What names are you thinking of giving your baby?

_____

_____

_____

_____

How do you feel now?

____ Excited

____ Scared

____ Happy

____ Depressed

____ A little bit of all of these

Other feelings? _____

_____

What are your special hopes? _____

_____

_____

Do you have new concerns now? _____

_____

_____

Share how you feel with your partner or husband, or with a close friend.

Chapter 10

Your Baby's Birth

By this time, you probably are very tired of being pregnant and ready to move on to parenthood. As you wait for childbirth to start, you may feel both excited and worried.

The natural way childbirth happens is amazing. If this is your first baby, it may seem very strange. Your body will take over and do what it needs to do. Learning about what will happen will make it less mysterious or scary.

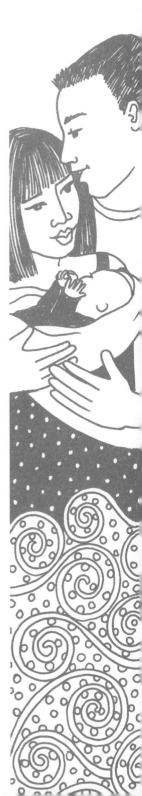

This chapter includes:

Be prepared, page 128

- What to take to the hospital
- Labor signs—When to call your health care provider
- Cesarean delivery
- Tips for your birth partner

Labor, page 136

- The stages of birth
- Timing your contractions
- Coping with pain during labor

Delivery, page 143

- What happens during delivery
- What happens right after delivery
- Birth record page

Be Prepared

This chapter gives you the facts of a normal birth. It is best to read it before your ninth month. To be completely ready, you will need to know more. Going to a childbirth class is the best way to learn what you and your partner can do to help delivery go well. If you have not been able to take a class, be sure to tell your doctor or nurse-midwife.

Information for the hospital or birth center

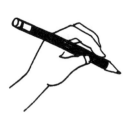

Collect this information ahead of time:

___ Blood type (ask your doctor or nurse) _____

___ Your doctor or nurse-midwife's name

_____

Phone number _____

___ The name of the baby's doctor or nurse practitioner (write inside the front cover, too)

_____

Phone number _____

___ Your insurance company or plan

_____

Your policy number _____

___ Do you plan to breastfeed? _____

___ Do you want to breastfeed right after birth?

_____

___ If your baby is a boy, do you want him circumcised before he goes home? _____

What should I take to the hospital?

Pack your bag several weeks before your due date. You need to be ready in case your baby comes early. Things to take:

___ This book

___ A watch with a second hand for timing your contractions. A pen or pencil and paper for making notes.

___ A CD, DVD, or iPod player and your favorite music. Soft, quiet music can help you relax during labor.

___ A camera to record the birth. If you want this, make sure you have film or the battery is charged. Test the camera ahead of time to make sure it is working properly.

___ Sugarless candies to keep your mouth moist

___ A nursing bra. A short robe, bed jacket, or sweater that opens in front, slippers, and warm socks, in case the hospital room is cool.

___ Hairbrush, toothbrush, toothpaste, makeup (Leave all jewelry and money at home.)

___ Money for your birth partner to use for coffee and meals

___ Snacks for your birth partner and for you after birth. Prunes, nuts, whole-wheat crackers, and apples will help keep your bowels moving. They also will be tastier than most hospital food.

___ Clothes for you to wear home. Choose something loose, even maternity clothes. Your body will need some time to return to your normal shape.

___ Clothes for your baby to wear home, such as a sleeper with legs. If it is cold, add a hat and thick blanket. (Clothes with legs are important, so the car seat harness will fit between your baby's legs.)

___ Car seat for your baby's first ride home. (Practice buckling it into the car ahead of time.) You and your baby must ride buckled up, even if you take a taxi. If you do not have a car seat by now, ask if the hospital has low-cost seats.

Preparing for labor

No one can tell exactly when your labor will begin. Labor will start when your baby and your body are ready. During the ninth month, your doctor or nurse-midwife will check often for changes in your cervix and the baby's position. Some women's bodies show clear signs before labor begins. Others do not.

Labor usually begins any time from two weeks before your due date to two weeks afterward. Labor may take a few hours or more than a day. First babies usually take longer than others.

Signs of labor

These are the main signs of labor, but you may not have all of them.

- A glob of thick mucus (mucous plug) with a little bright red blood in your underpants.

- Bag of waters breaks—Clear liquid that gushes or leaks from your vagina. It may break up to a day before labor starts or only after contractions begin. (Call right away when this happens.)

- Contractions that get stronger, last longer, and come closer and closer together. They get stronger when you move around. Write down on page ___ how long they last and how often they come. Your doctor or nurse midwife will want to know this.

- Pain or tightening of muscles that starts in your lower back and moves around to your belly.

- Several soft bowel movements.

If your baby is late

Your baby is not really late until two weeks after his due date. This may seem like a very long time to wait, but remember, no one is pregnant forever!

If you have not started labor one or two weeks after the baby was due, your doctor or nurse-midwife will help get labor started.

When to call the doctor or midwife

If you are not sure when to call, do so when:

- Your bag of water breaks.
- Your contractions have come about 5 to 10 minutes apart for at least an hour.
- You cannot walk or talk during contractions.

Tell your provider as much as you can about what is happening to you.

Call any time, day or night. It is better to call early rather than wait too long. You may be told to stay at home for a while longer. This is most likely if this is your first birth.

False labor

Sometimes it is hard to tell if your contractions are "real." Signs of false labor:

- Contractions do not get stronger and longer when you move or walk. They may stop completely in a few hours.
- Contractions go away when you drink several glasses of water.

Walk around and time the contractions. If they keep going or you are not sure, call your doctor or nurse midwife. She will not mind being called at any time. Sometimes the only way to know if true labor has started is to be checked by your provider. She can tell how much your cervix has effaced and dilated.

Sudden, unexpected delivery

Sometimes a baby might start to come out before his mother can get to the hospital or birth center. See the next page for some tips if this happens to you. This information is no substitute for help from paramedics or instructions from a health care provider by telephone.

- Call 911 right away if your baby starts to come out before you get to the hospital. Paramedics know how to deliver babies. You also can call the hospital's birth center or your doctor or nurse-midwife for help.

- Do not try to drive to the hospital. If you are in the car, stop in a safe place.

- If the baby comes out before medical help arrives, clean his face and dry his head. Do not pull on or cut the cord.

- Lay the baby on your chest against your skin. Cover both of you with a coat or sweater. Cover your baby's head to keep him warm.

- Breastfeed your baby.

- Push out the placenta. Keep it for the doctor.

- Get medical help as soon as possible.

Inducing labor

Sometimes it is necessary to make labor start (induce labor). This is done most often if labor has not started by two weeks after your due date. It can also be done if problems come up earlier or sometimes for non-medical reasons.

Labor can be started with drugs or by using measures such as breaking the amniotic sac. The doctor or nurse-midwife decides what to do by checking your cervix. It is best if the cervix is soft and has started to dilate and efface.

Inducing labor does not always work. If that is the case, a cesarean section would be done.

Cesarean delivery

It is important for any woman to be aware that a cesarean section might be needed. The health care provider may plan to do it if he knows that you or your baby has a medical problem that makes vaginal birth unwise. This could be because of twins or multiples or a problem with your baby. It could be because you have a medical condition such as preeclampsia or sores from genital herpes.

A C-section also may be done if problems come up during labor or delivery. Some of those problems would be:

- The baby is turned bottom down (breech) or sideward instead of head down and cannot be turned.
- Active labor has stopped (labor is not "progressing"), even after trying non-surgical measures.
- The baby is too large to fit through your pelvis.
- There are problems with the umbilical cord or placenta.
- The baby is not doing well during labor.

There are some risks from a C-section. Your health or that of your baby would be worth the risk.

A C-section usually takes less than an hour. The baby is born in the first 10 minutes. It is often done with a spinal anesthetic, so you can be awake during the operation.

Vaginal birth after cesarean

If you are trying a vaginal birth after a C-section, your health care provider will watch your condition closely. There is a small risk that the scar in the uterus might break where the earlier cut was made. Your health care provider will know as your labor progresses if vaginal birth will work. If it is not going well, you will be given another C-section.

Tips for a birth partner

Here are ways to help both at home and after you get to the hospital or birth center.

- **Keep calm** and cheerful. Help your partner breathe and relax during contractions.
- Time her contractions so she will know what progress she is making. (See page 138.)

- Play favorite CDs or a radio softly if music relaxes her.

- **Keep the room quiet** while your partner is having contractions. If visitors are distracting, ask them to leave the room for a while. This is not a good time for chatting.

- **Encourage her to change positions** or walk around. Even if she doesn't want to move, it could help her be more comfortable.

  - Massage her back lightly to help her relax during contractions. Press on her lower back firmly if it aches. Ask her what helps the most.

  - Urge her to rest between contractions. Help her breathe calmly during the contractions.

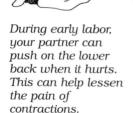

During early labor, your partner can push on the lower back when it hurts. This can help lessen the pain of contractions.

- **Try to stay calm** even if it upsets you to see your partner in pain or her body working so hard. It is normal for her to have nausea and pain. Remind her (and yourself) that the hardest part will be over soon.

- If you feel tired, take a few minutes away by yourself. Leave the room, get a snack, or go outside into the fresh air. You will be more able to help if you are not exhausted.

As a father, you play a very important part of the birth of your baby. Being there to comfort your partner and welcome your child into the world is very special.

- **Speak up** if you think your partner is having problems that are unusual. Ask the nurse to check her.

- Ask questions if the doctor or nurse midwife thinks your partner needs some kind of medication or a change in the birth plan.

If you are helping as a friend, you probably will always have a special feeling for this baby.

As a birth partner, do not be shy about asking questions. Make sure that both of you understand what is happening. If the doctor or nurse midwife thinks it is necessary to do something that you did not expect, ask him to explain. Make sure you understand why these things are needed before anything is done.

The Stages of Birth

In the last few weeks before the birth, the uterus drops (sinks down) between the pelvic bones. Even before labor begins, Braxton-Hicks contractions press the baby down against the cervix. The cervix starts softening and changing shape. It gets thinner (effaces) and opens (dilates) as the baby moves down.

These are the stages of birth:

1. **Labor:** Opening of the cervix. Regular contractions pull the cervix open. You need to try to relax as much as possible. This will help control pain.

2. **Birth of the baby:** The baby moves through the open cervix, into the birth canal. The vagina and perineum stretch wide open and the baby is born. You help by pushing with the contractions.

3. **Delivery of the placenta:** The placenta comes off the wall of the uterus and comes out. You may need to push a few more times.

4. **Recovery:** The uterus starts to shrink while you rest and start to relax.

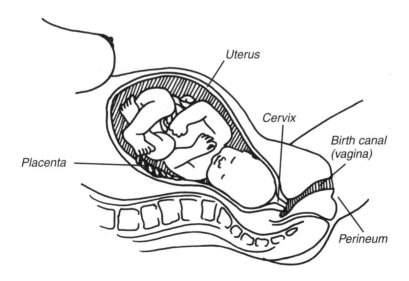

Parts of your body involved with birth

STAGE 1: Labor

During pregnancy, the uterus has grown into the largest, strongest muscle in your body. When labor starts, it contracts without any help from you. This can seem very strange at first.

Your job will be to help the uterus by letting it do its work. You help by relaxing as much as you can during contractions and resting between contractions. You can help by staying somewhat active, such as walking around. Lying down can slow labor. Avoid pushing during this time. Pushing can slow the opening of the cervix.

Contractions do the work

In labor, your uterus is working to dilate the cervix. Relax and let the uterus do what it is made to do.

How your cervix opens during the first stage:

Medical professionals measure these changes in centimeters instead of inches.

- **Early labor:** Contractions are short and not very strong. Your cervix opens to 4 centimeters.* You can relax at home during this time.

- **Active labor:** Contractions are longer and stronger. They come closer together. During this time you should go to the birth center or hospital. Your cervix will open to 8 centimeters.

- **Transition:** Contractions now are hardest, strongest, and come closest together. The cervix dilates completely, from 8 to 10 centimeters. (4 inches). This is wide enough for your baby's head to go through.

Early labor

Early labor can take a few hours or a few days. You will be more comfortable at home at this time. There is no need to be in the hospital or birth center until you are in active labor. Getting to the hospital early does not help your baby come quicker.

Check back to page 130 for signs of labor and when to call your doctor or nurse-midwife. Also, call

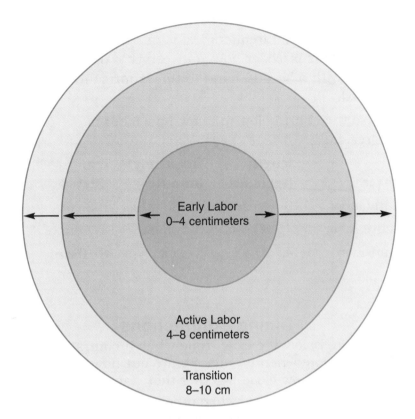

Early Labor
0–4 centimeters

Active Labor
4–8 centimeters

Transition
8–10 cm

The real size of your cervix as it opens around your baby's head!

your health care provider if anything unusual happens or if you have questions.

While you are in early labor, you can do some normal things, like cooking, taking walks, and visiting with friends. Eat lightly and drink water or juice. Try to relax but do not simply lie down. Sitting up, standing, and walking help the baby move down into the birth canal.

When a contraction happens, practice breathing and relaxation exercises you have learned. Start timing your contractions so you will know when to call the health care provider.

Keep track of your contractions

The length and frequency of your contractions tell you and your provider how your cervix is dilating. Use a watch with a second hand to time your contractions (see box).

Use the chart below to know how labor is progressing.

*Frequency:
How often the contractions start. Measure the amount of time there is between the beginning of one contraction and the beginning of the next one.

Phase	length (seconds)	frequency* (minutes)	cm. dilated
Early labor	30-45 sec.	15-30 min.	0-3 cm.
Active labor	45-60 sec.	3-5 min.	4-7 cm.
Transition	45-90 sec.	2-3 min	8-10 cm.

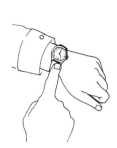

Timing Contractions

Write below the exact time when a contraction begins. Note when it ends. Figure out how longs it lasted and how close together they happen.

Also note the time when other signs happen. The waters may break during this time, for example.

Time Started	Time ended	Number of seconds contraction lasted	Frequency of contractions	Other Signs*
_____	_____	_____	_____	_____
_____	_____	_____	_____	_____
_____	_____	_____	_____	_____
_____	_____	_____	_____	_____
_____	_____	_____	_____	_____
_____	_____	_____	_____	_____
_____	_____	_____	_____	_____
_____	_____	_____	_____	_____
_____	_____	_____	_____	_____
_____	_____	_____	_____	_____
_____	_____	_____	_____	_____

(Use another piece of paper to continue your notes.)

Active labor

Once you have arrived at the hospital or birth center and been checked in, a labor and delivery nurse will help you know what to do. The nurses or your nurse-midwife will have many practical suggestions. They have helped many women through labor. Their advice about positions, activities, and breathing can be very helpful. Make sure they also have your birth plan.

Be sure to drink liquids or suck on ice chips to keep from getting dehydrated. Urinate whenever you need to.

It will be easier to relax in a quiet, peaceful room. If people in the hall or visitors distract you, you can close the door or ask people to wait outside.

Most mothers do not go through labor lying down. Other positions often help women feel more comfortable. They also can help birth go quicker or easier.

Some positions to try:

- Walking
- Standing leaning forward against your partner
- Resting on hands and knees
- Squatting and leaning back with support

Straight talk about pain

The pain of childbirth is natural, "good pain." There is no need to be afraid of it. It comes from the hard work your uterus is doing. It also comes from the stretching of the cervix, vagina, and perineum. It will be almost gone as soon as your baby is born.

You may want the good feeling of giving birth without drugs. If your labor is going well, you may only need the relaxation methods and other remedies listed on page 140.

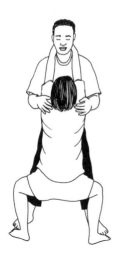

How to reduce pain naturally

- Have a birth partner and/or a doula to support and encourage you.
- Use breathing and massage methods to relax.
- Walk slowly with your partner holding you.
- Try different positions—sit upright, squat, kneel on hands and knees, sit on a birthing ball.
- Soak in a warm (not hot) bathtub—after you are at least 5 cm dilated. Some hospitals and birth centers have tubs in birth rooms.

Back pain

Back pain often happens when the baby is positioned with the back of his head toward your back. (Most have their face toward the back during labor.) This position makes the head push against the bones of your lower back. These are some ways to lessen back pain:

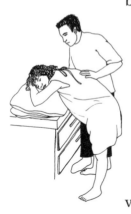

- Have your partner massage or press against your lower back.
- Lean forward against your partner or a table, or on a birthing ball.
- Lay cold packs on your lower back.
- Take a warm shower with water spraying on your lower back.

However, if labor is very long or contractions are very hard, you may want some pain medication. You should not feel that you have failed if you decide to use pain medication. One person may be able to bear much more pain than another.

Drugs have limits

There is no way to have a completely pain-free delivery. Even if you want pain medications, you will have to cope with pain without drugs during early labor. Sometimes there might not be time for the medication to take effect or some reason why certain medications cannot be given. So it is important to know how to relax to handle pain.

Different kinds of drugs can be used depending on:

- Your condition
- The condition of your baby
- What progress you have made in labor

Most drugs have some side effects. Some of those effects are rare but serious. It is important to know about these before you start labor, when it may be hard to think and make decisions. Learn about the different kinds of pain relief you can use and their side effects.

Kinds of pain medication

At a prenatal checkup, ask your health care provider about the kinds of drugs she prefers to use and why. Think about the benefits and side effects. None of these are given during early labor.

These drugs usually are very safe. However, it is important to know the risks before you agree to use any drug.

- **Pain relievers,** like Demerol, are narcotics. They lessen pain but do not block it completely. These drugs can affect the newborn baby's breathing if given late in labor. They can make you feel dizzy, or confused, or like throwing up.

- **Tranquilizers** may help if you are very nervous and other relaxation methods have not worked. You can feel contractions. They may be given with narcotics. These drugs may affect the new baby as well as the mother.

- **A spinal or epidural block** numbs the lower part of your body. Drugs given through a very narrow tube put into the space around your spinal cord in the lower part of your back (see picture). You feel very little or no pain.

  After the tube is put in place, you will not be able to walk, change positions, or take a warm

Putting the tube for the epidural into the space around the spinal cord. The lower body (shaded) will be numb.

bath. You can still push during the second stage of labor, but the nurse may have to tell you when the contractions are happening.

In some cases, an epidural makes labor go quicker. In other cases, labor may take longer. There sometimes are after-effects for the mother, such as severe headache. It has fewer effects on the newborn than other kinds of drugs.

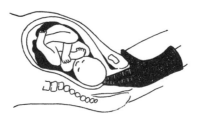

1. The first stage: Labor
The cervix has thinned out and opened. The baby starts to move into the vagina. In most cases a baby is born head first.

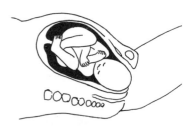

2. The second stage: Delivery
Now the baby's head has reached the opening of the vagina. The skin around the vagina stretches. If it does not stretch enough, an episiotomy may be done.

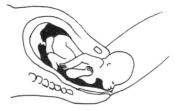

3. The baby's head appears. The shoulders come next. After that, the rest of the body slips out very quickly.

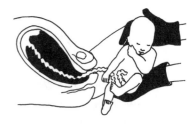

4. Now the newborn baby begins to breathe and is checked quickly. The umbilical cord will be clamped and cut. The placenta is delivered after more contractions.

A vaginal birth

STAGE 2: Delivery of your baby

After the cervix is completely open, you will be able to push your baby through the birth canal and out. You will feel like you should push (bear down) during contractions. This urge to push may feel like needing to have a bowel movement.

"I gave birth to my second baby standing up. It was much more comfortable than lying on my back."

While you push, hold your breath only for short periods. Take several quick breaths while pushing. Rest between contractions.

This stage can take some time. Your nurse-midwife or labor nurse will be with you. She will check on how far down the baby is moving. Your vagina will slowly stretch as the baby moves into it. Every push helps open the birth canal.

When the baby's head is all the way down the birth canal, the perineum must stretch wide enough to make way for the baby's head. You may have a burning feeling as the head presses against the skin.

At times, your doctor or nurse-midwife may ask you not to push hard. This gives the perineum time to stretch. This can help avoid cutting the perineum (an episiotomy). She may hold her hand on the top of the baby's head to slow down delivery. Warm towels or gentle massage may also be used to help avoid tearing. However, it may be necessary to do an episiotomy.

Sometimes a baby's head is not coming out as it should. The doctor may use forceps or a vacuum extractor to gently pull it out.

After the head has been born, the rest of your baby's body slips out very fast. You will feel a great relief that delivery is almost over! Contractions may continue, but they will be much more gentle.

Your baby may be placed right on your abdomen, skin to skin. He may be wrapped up to keep warm while you hold him.

STAGE 3: Delivery of the placenta

The delivery of the placenta, sometimes called the "afterbirth," will seem easy. Your uterus will contract a few more times. You may need to push a little more to help the placenta come out. The health care provider will check to make sure all of it has been delivered.

STAGE 4: Beginning of recovery

Now you can relax. You can cuddle your baby and breastfeed for the first time. You can eat, drink some water or juice, and relax.

If you had an episiotomy or tear, it will be sewn up. Your vaginal area will be cleaned up. You will be given a pad to wear to absorb any blood.

During this stage, your nurse or nurse-midwife will feel your abdomen often. She is checking your uterus to make sure it is contracting. The nurse may massage the top of the uterus to make it contract. You may be able to massage it yourself. It should feel hard and be about the size of a grapefruit. Touch it yourself to feel how it is changing.

These contractions can be uncomfortable but are normal and will limit bleeding. Sometimes medication is given to help the uterus stay firm.

Welcome your new baby!

Your new baby has come into the world. He may look strange to you at birth. He will be wet, and his skin will be a blue-purple color. He may be covered with white vernix and streaks of blood.

Your baby may seem lifeless for a moment, but after his first breath he may begin to cry. His lungs are taking in air for the first time. His skin will start to turn pink or reddish, closer to its natural color. The doctor or nurse-midwife may suck mucus out of his nose and mouth to help him breathe better.

The umbilical cord will be clamped and cut. This separates your baby from your body. Your birth partner may be able to cut it if he wants. Cutting the cord does not hurt you or your baby.

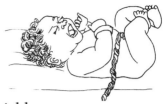

Your baby's general health will be checked quickly one minute and five minutes after birth. Your doctor or nurse midwife will look at his heart rate, breathing, muscles, body reflexes, and skin color.

After a few minutes, the nurse will clean up the baby and will measure him. She will put on a tiny diaper and cap. Then she will swaddle him snugly. Now you can hold him as long as you want. He may want to breastfeed now.

This can be a very emotional time. Some women may feel overwhelming love for their babies right away. Others can't believe the birth has really happened. Some may wonder if they can take care of such a small person. All of these feelings are normal at this time.

You or your partner may want to write notes about your baby's birth on the next page. This will help you remember this special day.

Birth Surprises

Preterm birth

A baby born earlier than 37 weeks is called preterm or premature (a "premie"). Twins and multiple babies often come early. A premature baby needs extra care after birth. Yet today, many very small premature babies grow up to be healthy people.

A premie who needs a lot of medical treatment may be taken to a special care nursery (newborn intensive care unit or NICU). This might be at another hospital. If this happens, try to spend as much time there as possible. Your baby needs to hear your voice and feel your touch even when he is very tiny.

Low birth-weight baby

Some babies born after 37 weeks are smaller than usual, under $5^1/_2$ pounds (2500 grams). These babies may be small because they have other health problems. They often need special care. As with premies, with good care, most will grow up to be healthy people.

Cesarean section

If you had not expected to have a cesarean, you may feel very upset or disappointed afterward. You may think you have failed. Try to remember that you did the best you could.

My Baby's Birth Day!

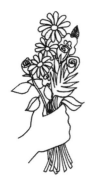

My baby's name is _____

Baby was born on _____ (date)
    at _____ time in the morning __ or night __.

Weight: _____ pounds

Length: _____ inches

Head size (distance around): ____ inches

First sign of labor: _____

Date and time when I arrived at the hospital or birth
    center _____

I was in labor for _____ hours.

Things I did that helped labor go well _____

_____

Pain medication I was given, if any _____

_____

Special things done by my doctor or nurse-midwife to
    help deliver my baby

_____

_____

_____

How I felt right after birth _____

_____

Comments by my birth partner _____

_____

Comments by my doctor or nurse-midwife

_____

_____

What happens next?

Now that your baby is born, you finally can see and hold him or her. What an exciting time! Take some time to hold your baby close right after birth. Most newborns are wide awake for about 1 to 2 hours after birth. Then they need a long sleep.

Now is a good time to start breastfeeding. The colostrum in your breasts gives him a good start. Let him feed before he gets sleepy.

Don't be surprised if your baby's head and nose look strange. This is from being squeezed through the birth canal. They will return to their normal shape in a day or two.

Soon after birth, your infant will be weighed and measured. He will be given an injection of vitamin K to prevent possible bleeding problems. Medicine will be put in his eyes to prevent infection. It may make his eyes red for a day or two.

Your nurse-midwife or hospital nurses will help you start to feed and care for your baby. Nurses are good teachers. Ask them any questions you have.

Coming home

If both you and your baby are doing well, you will probably go home within a day or two after delivery. If you have had a cesarean delivery you will need to stay longer to recover. If your baby is very small or had problems at birth, he will probably stay longer than you do.

A home visit from a nurse can be very helpful to new parents. If your hospital or health plan does not offer you this service, ask if you can have a home visit.

Your health care provider, your baby's doctor or nurse practitioner, and the hospital or birth center all have people who can help you, day or night.

Put a picture of your
new baby or your baby
and family tree

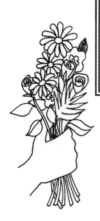

Chapter 11

Basics of Newborn Care

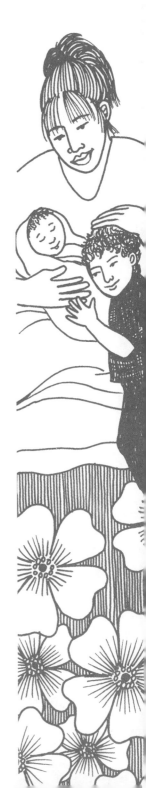

New baby care is very basic: keep your baby warm, fed, comforted, and clean. It may take a little practice to get good at doing these things. Your baby will survive while you learn. The nurse, midwife, or doula will help you learn these basics before you take your baby home.

The most important thing is to be gentle and loving with your baby. The other important thing is to get as much rest as possible, so your body can heal. Ask others to do some things to help you, such as laundry, cooking, shopping for groceries, and housecleaning.

See Chapter 15 for Warning Signs to Know.

See Chapter 12 for details about feeding your baby.

This chapter includes:
- What your baby looks like
- What your baby can do

The first day basics, page 151
- Holding and carrying your baby
- Diapering and bathing
- Dressing your baby

Care for a baby with a special need, page 161

What your newborn looks like

A baby who has just been born looks very different from a baby who is even a month old. A normal newborn will change a lot in the first few weeks.

Your baby's face may seem puffy. Her eyelids may be swollen from eye medicine given to all newborns. Her eyes may seem to look in different directions. If you had a vaginal delivery, her head is likely to be cone-shaped and her nose flattened. This is from being squeezed coming through the birth canal.

Your baby's skin may have a reddish color, with little white spots (milia) on her nose, cheeks, and chin. The white coating on her skin at birth may stay in the folds of her skin. She may have fine, soft hair in her back and face (lanugo). Lanugo is found mainly on premature babies. Her skin may be dry and peeling. This is most likely in babies born late.

Her head will have two soft spots called fontanels. They are places where the bones of her skull have not grown together yet. You can feel a large one is on the top and a small one on the back. The fontanels will close slowly by about 18 months of age. For now, a strong layer under the skin protects her brain.

What can a newborn do?

Your baby can see things close to her. She will be able to see your face when you hold her. She can hear and likes calm, soft, high voices. She can taste and smell.

Your new baby's body moves automatically in some ways. These are called reflexes. They will disappear as she develops. You will see her:

- Turn her head and open her mouth (called "rooting") if you stroke her cheek
- Startle (jump, act surprised) when she hears a loud sound.
- Hold your finger tightly when you touch her palm
- Lift up one foot if you hold her up with her feet touching a surface

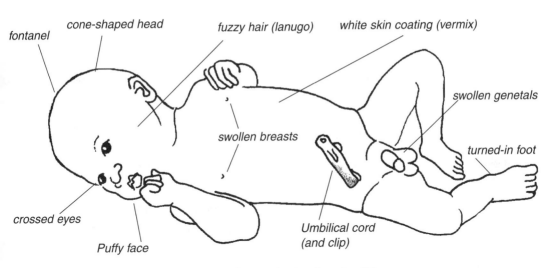

fontanel

cone-shaped head

fuzzy hair (lanugo)

white skin coating (vermix)

swollen genetals

swollen breasts

turned-in foot

crossed eyes

Umbilical cord
(and clip)

Puffy face

What a newborn baby looks like

The first day

Feeding your newborn

Your baby knows how to suck, so offer her your breast right after birth. Many babies are very alert for the first couple of hours and then fall asleep. She may be ready to latch on right away. During the first day or two, she may not be very hungry. It is normal if she does not want to breastfeed (nurse) very often at this time.

The most important things about breastfeeding are:

- Holding your baby so her tummy is facing your chest.

- Making sure her mouth is wide open and her lips out, so she gets part of the areola (dark area around the nipple) into her mouth with the nipple.

- Avoiding giving water or formula in a bottle, which make her less hungry for breast milk.

The nurses or a breastfeeding expert (lactation specialist) will help you get started. If you have questions, be sure to ask before you go home. If problems come up after you go home, call right away for advice.

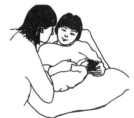

A lactation specialist can help you get started with breastfeeding.

If you have decided not to breastfeed, give only very small amounts of formula at first. Newborns have very small stomachs and may not seem very hungry.

For many important details on feeding, read Chapter 12.

Holding and comforting her

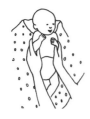

Babies love to be held, rocked, and walked. They love movement. Walking and rocking give babies the same motion they felt in the uterus.

Cuddle your baby against your chest so she can hear your heart beat, feel your warmth, and smell the scent of your body. Stroke her body.

Talk to her in a soft voice. Babies like high, singsong sounds. Try not to feel silly talking this way—it is natural. You can use real words, not just "baby talk."

Sucking is comforting to a baby even when she is not hungry. Wash your hands and let her suck on your little finger.

Your baby probably will like being swaddled, wrapped snugly in a thin blanket (see pictures). This makes her feel secure, the way she was contained in your uterus. Watch how the nurse wraps the blanket around and tucks it in.

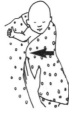 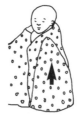 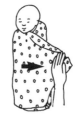 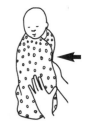

1. Place baby's head at one corner of a receiving blanket.

2. Then wrap one corner around and tuck it in.

3. Pull the bottom corner up to her chest.

4. Finally, wrap the other corner over her arms.

5. Tuck corner of blanket under your baby.

Swaddling your baby

When your baby cries, try to figure out what she is telling you. Is she hungry, wet, tired, or lonely? You will learn how to know what she needs. She may just want to be cuddled. Walking slowly with her in your arms is very soothing.

Your new baby may like being held with her skin against your bare chest, with a light blanket over both of you. This is called kangaroo care. It is especially good for premature newborns and can help them grow well.

For many details on behavior, read Chapter 13.

First Steps of Baby Care

Keep her warm

New babies are used to the warmth of your body. Keep your baby's body covered lightly indoors. Use a little cap to keep her from losing heat through her head during the first few days. However, do not cover her with too many layers unless the room is very cool or you are going outside in cool weather. She could get a fever if covered with too many blankets.

How can you tell if your baby is warm enough? Her back and tummy should feel warm like your body but not hot or sweaty. It is normal for a baby's hands and feet to feel cool.

Keep her clean

Change your baby's diaper often to protect her tender skin. Some babies cry when they are being changed because they feel cold when they are naked. Be sure to wash your hands well with soap before and after.

It is good to check her diaper often. Wet diapers tell you she is getting enough breast milk or formula. After feeding is going well, she should have at least 6 to 8 wet diapers each day.

Keep germs away

Wash your hands often when caring for your baby. Make sure that others who care or play with her also wash their hands first. Even if hands look clean, they can carry germs.

Keep your new baby away from people with colds or other illnesses she might catch. It is best not to take your baby into crowds, such as stores or parties, until she is older. This is especially important if she is a premie or has any breathing problems.

For important details on baby care, read later pages in this chapter.

Keeping your baby safe

The two most important safety concerns with new babies are Sudden Infant Death syndrome (SIDS) and car crash injury.

Sleep safety basics:
* Always put your baby to sleep on her back unless there is a medical reason to lay her on her tummy.

* Have her sleep in the same room with you but in her own crib.

* Use a firm mattress and keep pillows and quilts out of the crib.

* Dress her warmly and keep the room comfortably cool. She should be warm but not hot.

* Keep her away from smoky places.

* Breastfeed her.

Car safety basics:
* Make sure to use a car seat on every car ride.

* Buckle the harness snugly over both shoulders and between her legs.

* Anchor the car seat tightly in the back seat, facing the back of the car.

For many important details about safety, read Chapter 14.

Watching for signs of health problems

Read Chapter 15, page 207 for signs of serious illness that you need to know. Be sure to call the nurse or doctor right away if your baby has any of them.

These things may never happen, but—if they do—you must be ready to take your baby to the doctor or nurse practioner.

Watch out for severe diarrhea, vomiting, or trouble breathing. You cannot wait for any of these problems to get better by themselves.

Before you take your baby home

- Make sure you know whom to call if you or your baby has health problems.

- Get the name and phone number of a breastfeeding consultant.

- Make sure your baby has started to breastfeed. Know how to hold her facing your breast. Practice squeezing (expressing) a small amount of milk out of your nipple with your fingers.

- Buckle your baby's car seat into the back seat for the ride home. Take off swaddling blankets before putting her in the car seat. Put a blanket over the harness if the weather is cold.

- Make an appointment to bring your baby to her doctor or nurse practitioner for her first checkup.

The first weeks at home

Holding and carrying your baby

Babies love to be held. Pick her up as often as she wants. You can't spoil her at this age by holding her too much.

Keep one hand behind your baby's head. A baby's head is heavy and her neck is not strong enough to hold it up. Hold her up on your shoulder, cradle her in one arm, or tuck her feet under your arm (football hold), always holding her head.

One way to have your baby close while you do other things is to use a sling or front-carrier. This makes it easy to take a walk, do light housework, or go shopping with your baby. This can be very soothing for a fussy baby or one that doesn't go to sleep easily.

Keeping baby clean

Baby's bowel movements

What goes in, must come out. All parents must deal with cleaning their baby's bottom, even though it may not be much fun.

Don't be surprised by your newborn's first few bowel movements (stool). They will be thick and black. The next few will be greenish. After that, they will be yellow. They will have very little smell until your baby begins eating solid foods.

Your baby's stools will look different depend on whether you feed her formula or breast milk.

- Breast-milk makes a light yellow, very soft stool, like lumpy mustard. In the early weeks, a baby may have 8 to10 small stools each day. Later, one stool each day or every few days is common.

- Formula makes a tan or yellow stool (about as firm as peanut butter). A baby will often have one or two movements each day.

If the stools get hard and dry, your baby may not be getting enough liquid. This also can happen if she has had vomiting or fever. Call your baby's doctor or nurse practitioner.

*Genitals: A boy's penis or a girl's vulva.

Cleaning your baby's genitals*

Baby wipes are handy but not necessary. You can use lukewarm water and cotton balls or washcloths. Wash with soap after bowel movements. Rinse and dry with clean cotton balls or cloths.

Always wipe your baby's genitals from front to back, whether you have a girl or a boy. This keeps germs in the stool from getting into the opening of your baby's genitals.

If your baby boy is not circumcised, don't try to pull the foreskin of his penis back. It will not become loose until about age 2.

A newborn girl may have some bloody or milky discharge from her vagina. This is normal in the first week.

Avoid using baby oil or powder. Although they are sold for babies, they can irritate the skin. Powder made with talc (talcum powder) can be very bad for a baby's lungs.

Care for a circumcised penis

A baby boy's circumcision can take one to two weeks to heal. While it is healing, wash the penis very gently every day. Drip warm soapy water gently over it. Rinse it by dripping warm clean water, and then very carefully pat it dry.

Ask your doctor or nurse practitioner if you need to use any ointment on the circumcision. If the penis has a plastic ring on it, do not use ointment. Let the ring fall off by itself.

Fasten diapers loosely. Do not lay your baby on his tummy until the penis has healed.

Call the doctor of nurse if you see bleeding, signs of infection (white pus, redness, swelling), or if your baby has a hard time urinating.

Preventing diaper rash*

It is easy to prevent diaper rash if you:

*Diaper rash:
A red, bumpy rash around the genitals and buttocks.

- Change your baby's diaper as soon as possible after each bowel movement and every two to three hours when it is wet.

- Dry the area well after changing the diaper.

- Let your baby lie without a diaper on for a while every day. The air helps prevent diaper rash. Lay her naked on her tummy on a waterproof pad covered with a diaper or towel.

If your baby gets diaper rash, be sure to change diapers often. Wash the area well with warm water and dry it. Let your baby lie with her bottom bare each day. Spread a baby ointment (such as A & D ointment or zinc oxide) on the rash when you change diapers. If it does not get better soon, call the doctor or nurse. It might be an infection.

Caring for the umbilical cord stump

Keep the stump clean and dry. Clean the stump and the area at its base with warm water once a day and if it gets stool on it. Some health care providers suggest using isopropyl alcohol* instead of water. Let the stump dry in the air and fold the top of her diapers down below it. The stump will get dry and black and fall off in one to two weeks. Never try to pull it off.

* **Isopropyl alcohol:** The kind of alcohol used to kill germs (not for drinking).

Call your baby's doctor or nurse if the skin around the stump gets red or pus starts oozing from the area. (A little bit of bleeding is normal when the stump falls off.)

Bathing your new baby

If you keep your baby's face, neck, cord, and genitals clean, she will need a bath only every few days. When she gets older, she may enjoy having a bath more often.

Some health care providers advise giving a sponge bath until the cord has fallen off. Also, if your baby has been circumcised, you may want to give sponge baths until his penis has healed. Ask your provider if he or she thinks sponge bathing is best.

Some babies, especially premies, may benefit from being bathed while they are swaddled. Basically, this allows a baby to be wrapped up and kept warm while parts of her body are exposed and washed one at a time. The baby could be put into the tub with a light blanket around her.

Getting ready for the bath

Make sure the room is warm. The kitchen sink is usually a good place to give the bath, because you can stand comfortably. Use a baby tub or put a foam insert or a soft towel in the bottom of the clean kitchen sink.

Collect all the things you need before you start the bath. This is easier than looking for things while your baby is wet and soapy. Have these things where you can reach them:

- Washcloth and plastic cup (to scoop water)
- Gentle soap without perfume, baby shampoo
- Several towels
- Fresh clothes
- Clean diaper

Giving a Sponge bath

Give your baby a sponge bath on a wide flat surface (counter or table) in a warm room. Gather all the things you need. Have two bowls of lukewarm water within reach. Put a little mild soap in one.

- Lay your baby on a clean towel.
- Wash and dry her face before undressing her unless the room is quite warm.
- Wash, rinse, and dry one part of her body at a time. Start with her face and finish with her bottom.
- Always keep one hand on her so she will not fall.
- Wash her hair with fresh water after her body is clean and she is swaddled in a towel.

Tub bathing

After the cord has healed (and the circumcision if your boy has been circumcised), you can wash your baby in a sink or small tub. Put two to three inches of lukewarm water in the tub. A foam pad will help keep her from slipping around too much.

- Have everything you will need nearby. Test the water with your elbow to make sure it is not hot.
- Hold your baby under the head and shoulders with one arm. Soap and rinse with the other hand.
- Never leave your baby alone in the bath—even for a moment! You must always hold up her head and shoulders. A baby can drown quickly and silently if left alone.

Babies do not need oil or powder on their skin after a bath. If you want to use powder, avoid using "Baby powder" or other products made with talc or cornstarch. These can cause health problems.

Cleaning gums and teeth

Your baby will not get her first teeth for at least a few months. Before they come in, it is good to wipe her gums with a soft cloth every day. This helps her get used to the feeling of having her teeth cleaned. Once her first teeth start coming in, continue to wipe them daily or use a very soft, baby tooth brush with no toothpaste. Avoid toothpaste until age 2, when you can start using a tiny amount of paste (the size of a piece of rice).

"My baby didn't like having his teeth brushed. I wish I had started wiping his gums earlier."

It is important to prevent tooth decay in baby teeth. Your baby needs those teeth for many things besides chewing food. They are necessary for learning to talk. They hold space in the gums for the second (adult) set of teeth.

Dressing for inside and outside

Unless she is premature, your baby needs to wear only a little warmer clothing than you do. Dress her in one layer more than you are wearing. During the first week or two cover her head with a little cap. That will help keep her from losing heat through her head. If the weather is very cold or hot, it is best to keep your baby inside for the first few weeks.

Heavy blankets can make your baby too hot. Unless your baby is very small (less than about 4 1/2 pounds) or is out in cold weather, she does not need to be covered with thick blankets. A warm hat can be very helpful, however, in cold weather.

Protect her from the sun

An infant can get sunburned very easily, whether her skin is light or dark. Keep her in the shade or lightly covered if she is outside on a bright day between 10 AM and 3 PM. The sun can burn even if there are light clouds or if there is bright sun on snow.

It is best not to use sunscreen for babies under 6 months of age. Cover your baby up instead. Dress her in clothes that cover her arms and legs. A hat with a wide brim will protect her face, ears, and neck.

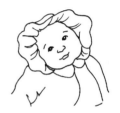

After the first six months, you can use an infant sunscreen with an SPF rating of 15 or higher. Keep it off her hands or other parts that she may put in her mouth.

When a baby needs special care

Some newborn babies have a birth defect or another health problem, like low birth weight or prematurity. Some of these problems can be explained, but others just happen. Some are more serious than others. If your baby has a special health care need, try not to blame yourself. It is best to focus on helping her get well and come home.

Your baby may need to stay in the hospital for medical care. She may be in the newborn intensive care unit (NICU or "nick-you") at a children's hospital. In the NICU, care is planned to help the baby feel comfortable, a little like being in the uterus. The lights are kept low. The room is as quiet as possible. Twins or multiples may be put in the same bed. This kind of care has been shown to help a baby develop as well as possible.

If possible, hold your baby by cuddling her skin-to-skin against your chest every day. This is called Kangaroo Care. Any new baby would like this! Dad's can do it too.

"When my baby was tiny, both her father and I loved holding her against our chests. She really seemed to like it too."

It is important for both you and your baby's father to be with your baby in the hospital as much as possible. She needs to hear your voices and feel your touch. This is just as important as all the tubes, machines, and medicines. Being with her will help her heal. Spending time with her will also help you learn how to care for her when she comes home.

Dealing with your feelings

If your child has a health problem at birth, it may be a big surprise for you. Parents whose baby is not born exactly the way they expected often feel very frightened, sad, guilty, or angry. These feelings are normal.

Here are some ways to cope:

- Spend as much time as possible with your baby.

- Try to be at the NICU when the doctor checks your baby every day, so you can ask questions. If there is something you do not understand, be sure to ask the health care professionals to explain.

- Find out as much as possible about your baby's condition. Ask the hospital social worker for help getting information. Look on the Internet.

- Ask for a second opinion from another doctor if you are not sure about approving any treatment.

- Talk with the social worker about your feelings. Partners may need support from professionals and other parents to get through this time. The social worker can link you with a parent support group.

Modern medical care helps many babies with special needs to lead healthy, happy lives. Your baby will need your love and attention. Caring for her can be very hard and very special at the same time.

See Chapter 15 for details to caring for a sick baby.

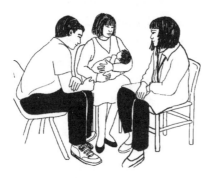

Chapter 12

Feeding Your Newborn

Your Most Important Task

Feeding time can be a calm, soothing time for you and your baby. Babies are happiest and grow best if they are fed whenever they show the first signs of hunger. When parents respond quickly to a baby's needs, the baby starts to learn to trust people. If a parent makes the baby wait, the baby learns that people may not help him.

Your baby needs more food some days than others. Feed him when he begins to act hungry. When he is growing faster, he will get hungry more often. A baby who is breastfeeding will suck more when he needs more. This makes the breasts produce more milk. If you are feeding formula to your baby, you will find

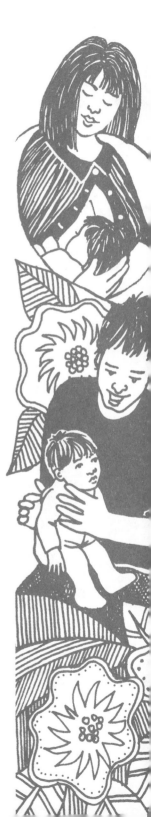

This chapter includes:

Basics of feeding your baby, page 164

- Hunger signs
- Signs your baby is getting enough milk

Breastfeeding basics, page 166

- Holding, latching on, help with problems

Bottle feeding basics, page 174

- Bottle feeding with breast milk or formula
- Feeding with formula

that he will take more at some feedings than others. Let him tell you how much he needs.

Basics for feeding

Learn the hunger signs

Try to feed your baby before he starts to cry. How can you tell that he is hungry? Watch for these signs:

- Sucking on his fist
- Making little soft sounds
- Turning his head toward your breast when you hold him

Some newborns are sleepy and need to be waked up to begin feeding. It is important for a new baby to go no more than two or three hours between feedings. You can wake him gently by changing his diaper, taking off some of his clothes, massaging his back, or holding him upright.

A special time

Feeding can take some time, so make sure you both are comfortable before you begin. Place a firm pillow in your lap to support your arm and your baby. This will help both of you to relax. Have a glass of water within reach. Listen to some slow, soft music.

Pay attention to your baby while you are feeding him. Turn your face toward him and smile. Talk softly or sing a quiet song. Take this time to help him feel secure and loved.

How do you know when he is full?

Babies usually know when they are full. At first, your baby's tummy is very small, so he will not be able to eat much at one feeding. Trying to make your baby to eat more than he wants is unhealthy for him and frustrating for both of you.

Watch for these signs so you can stop feeding when he has had enough.

- He stops sucking and doesn't need to burp.
- He turns his head away from the breast (or pushes the bottle away).
- He starts to fall asleep.

If your baby gets sleepy after only a few minutes of feeding, help him wake up. Hold him up, burp him, or change his diaper. Then offer him the nipple again.

Is your baby getting enough to eat?

Feed your baby as much as he wants when he is hungry. Here are some signs that he is getting enough:

- He has at least six to eight wet diapers every 24 hours. His bowel movements should be soft.
- He is gaining weight. (It is normal to lose weight during the first week after birth).
- He is sleepy or peaceful after eating and burping.

A baby under 6 months of age should get enough food from the breast or bottle. He should not need any other food.

It is hard to tell if a disposable diaper is wet. You can tell by holding it up to the light and comparing it to a dry one. You also can put a piece of tissue in the diaper. The tissue will stay wet.

Burping is part of feeding

Babies usually swallow some air when they are feeding. They often need to burp in the middle of a feeding and at the end.

Hold your baby on your shoulder, across your knees, or on your lap. Pat or rub his back gently for a few minutes. Some milk may come up with the burp. This is normal, so have an extra diaper handy to protect your clothes.

Warning: If your baby vomits forcefully, so liquid shoots several feet out of his mouth, he might have a serious problem. Call the doctor or nurse right away.

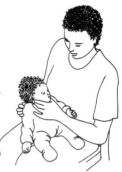

Burping a new baby

If you are feeding formula to your baby go to page 174.

Breastfeeding: Getting started

Breast milk is specially made for babies. It is the perfect food for the first year of life. The milk your breasts make during the first few days is especially nutritious. Breast milk changes as your baby's needs change. (For more about why breastfeeding is important for your baby, see Chapter 6.)

A baby does not need other foods until 5 to 6 months of age. Wait until he shows interest in them and can sit up and swallow well. The Academy of Pediatrics recommends feeding only breast milk for at least the first 6 months.

Most babies are ready to breastfeed right after birth. Many moms love nursing their babies during the first hour or two after birth. However, medicines given to some moms during labor and delivery may make their baby sleepy or not interested in eating during the first day. If this happens, don't worry. Your baby will be hungry soon.

If breastfeeding is not easy to you and your baby at first, you can learn how to make it work. As you both get used to breastfeeding, it will be easier.

Be sure to get help right away if you have any concerns (see below). Usually there is an answer.

Learning to breastfeed

How can you learn? If you have friends who have nursed their babies, you probably have seen how they do it. If not, or if you and your baby have trouble getting started, there are people who can help you. The nurses in the hospital or birth center will be eager to help you get started.

Ask your doctor or nurse-midwife for the name and phone number of a lactation consultant. You will have someone to call if you have any questions or problems after you leave the hospital. Lactation (breastfeeding) consultants are nurses or others with special training and experience with many nursing moms. Consultants who are certified use these initials, IBCLC, after their names.

You also can call a local member of an international breastfeeding group, La Leche League (see Chapter 17). Members are women who have nursed their babies. They can give you their wisdom and support.

Your breasts

Your breasts will be larger when they are making milk regularly. Your nipple and areola may also be larger.

Inside your breasts are the glands that make milk. They will feel like lumps all around your breast area. You may even feel them near your armpits. Tubes (ducts) carry the milk from the glands to your nipples.

After your baby starts sucking, you probably will be able to feel the breasts "let down." That happens when the milk (called hind milk) starts to flow from the glands. That milk is richer that what comes out in the first few minutes. It is important to let your baby suck as much on each breast as possible, so that he gets the hind milk. This also is important when pumping your breasts.

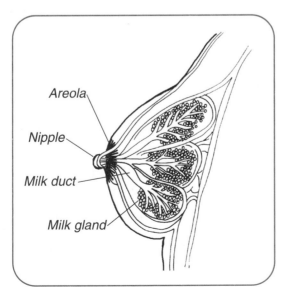

When your milk "comes in"

During the first few days, your breasts will make colostrum, the first milk, that is rich in antibodies. It is clear or yellowish.

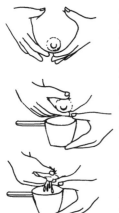

After two or three days, your breasts begin to fill with milk. This milk is thin and bluish. At this time, your breasts will get hard and painful (engorged) naturally. Nurse as often as possible to make your breasts feel better. Put warm cloths on your breasts or massage them before nursing to help the milk flow easier. They will only be engorged for a few days. After that, your breasts still will be large but not painful, unless you stop nursing suddenly.

If your areola gets so hard that your baby can't get it into his mouth, express (squeeze) a little milk out by hand. This will make the nipple softer. Massage or press on your breast firmly with your fingers from all sides toward the areola. Then hold your thumb above and fingers below and squeeze and release the areola.

Expressing breast milk by hand.

Basics of happy breastfeeding

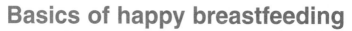

Breastfeeding may not come naturally to you, but almost any woman can do it. Once you get started, it usually is a very happy experience.

Follow these basic steps:

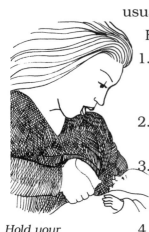

1. Hold your baby so his tummy faces your body. His head should face the nipple, so he doesn't have to turn his head to reach it.

2. Hold your breast outside the areola with your thumb on top.

3. Get your baby to open his mouth wide by touching his lower lip with your nipple. Try opening your mouth—he may do it too.

4. When he opens his mouth wide, pull him toward you. Guide the nipple and areola deeply into his mouth.

Hold your breast and pull him to it when he opens his mouth.

5. Make sure he pulls part of the areola into his mouth. Sucking only on the nipple will not work. Make sure his lower lip is out and the tip of his nose touches your breast. He still should be able to breathe.

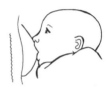

Baby's lower lip should be turned out.

6. Make sure he is swallowing. He will not swallow every time he sucks. You may hear him gulp or see small little movements of the skin in front of his ears.

If your nipples start to get sore, check:

- Your baby is lying facing your chest

- His head is not turned to the side

- He has only the nipple and part of the areola in his mouth.

Ways to hold your baby for breastfeeding

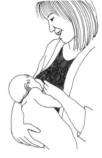

- Cradle position: Sit up straight in an armchair. Hold your baby across your chest. His head should be in the bend of your arm. Put a firm pillow under your baby's body and your elbow.

Cradle position

- Football position: Sit in a chair and hold your baby under your arm on a pillow. His head will be at your breast and his feet will be behind you. This is the most comfortable way to nurse if you have had a cesarean delivery.

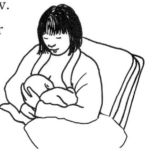

- Side-lying position: Lie in bed on your side. Your baby lies next to you on the mattress or in the bend of your elbow.

Football position

In all these positions, use pillows to make yourself and your baby comfortable. Double check that your baby's tummy is facing your body.

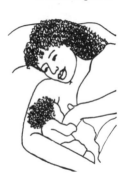

Side-lying position

Breastfeeding details

- After the first day, a baby under 2 months old needs to nurse every one to three hours or at least eight to twelve times in 24 hours. Some may eat more often during one part of the day than another.

- If your baby sleeps for more than four hours, it is important to wake him up gently to feed.

- If your nipple does not stand out very far, you can roll or pull it between your fingers before feeding. Your baby's sucking will pull it out of the areola.

- Switch breasts half way through each feeding when his sucking slows, after about 10 to 15 minutes. Start the next feeding with the breast he used last.

- If your baby stops nursing, he may simply need to burp. Hold him up and pat his back. Then offer him more from that breast or the other one.

- To get him to let go of the nipple, put your finger gently into the corner of his mouth. This will break the suction without hurting your nipple.

Is your baby getting enough breast milk?

Your breasts make just enough milk for your baby's needs. When he is hungry, he will suck more and they will make more milk. They can make enough to feed twins! Every few weeks your baby will have a growth spurt. This means he will nurse more often for a couple of days. This will increase your milk supply. It does not mean you cannot make enough milk.

To know your baby is getting enough to eat, make sure he is nursing often and well and seems to be happy after nursing. He should wet his diaper at least 8 times each day. Check it often if you are concerned.

Pacifiers and bottles for breastfed newborns

Avoid giving your baby a pacifier or a bottle of water or formula while he is learning to nurse. Here is why:

- Sucking builds up your supply of breast milk.

- Formula or water can take away his appetite for breast milk.

- A bottle or pacifier nipple is very different from your nipples. Milk flows out of a bottle much easier. Your baby may start to like the bottle better.

Many babies love to suck when they are not hungry. It is best to offer only your breast or your clean finger at first. Pacifiers can be used after your baby is nursing well. This is often between 4 and 6 weeks of age.

Twins and breastfeeding

You can breastfeed your twins. You may want to feed your newborns one at a time at first. As you and the babies get used to nursing, you can feed both at once. This will save you a lot of time. Some moms with twins or triplets breastfeed for at least a few months. Then they start offering some bottle feedings with breast milk or formula.

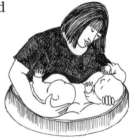

Get help for problems right away

If you are having a problem with nursing, ask for help now. Do not simply stop breastfeeding or wait until it gets worse. Call your doctor or nurse midwife, a breastfeeding consultant, WIC nurse, or a La Leche League group member for advice. They can give you practical tips and support to help with most problems.

Common problems that you should call about:

- Cracked or sore nipples

- A hard, red area of your breast that feels warm

- A very sleepy baby who does not wake for feedings

- Less than six wet diapers in 24 hours—after your milk comes in

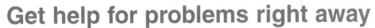

Delays in starting to breastfeed

Sometimes a mother and baby cannot begin nursing after delivery because of an illness or medical problem. Usually, a baby can begin breastfeeding later. He can be given the mom's breast milk from a bottle for a few days or even a few weeks. Even if your baby must be given formula for a short time, it is often possible for him to learn to nurse later.

If you cannot start nursing right after birth, talk to the nurse in the hospital or your nurse midwife as soon as possible. They can help you pump your breasts until your baby can nurse. Your milk is best—even during the first few days of life. Also, if you do not pump your breasts, they will stop making milk. You will not be able to start again later.

Giving vitamins or other supplements?

Ask your baby's doctor or nurse practitioner about giving your baby vitamin D and fluoride. Breast milk does not contain much of these things. In every other way, breast milk is the only food your baby needs now. After 6 months, your baby may need extra iron.

Caring for your breasts

Soon after birth, your breasts will fill with milk. They will swell and get hard (engorgement). This is natural but can be painful for a few days. Engorgement also can happen if you miss a feeding or stop nursing suddenly.

Your breasts will feel better as your baby starts sucking well and empties them often. After you have been breastfeeding for a few days, they will get softer and will stop hurting. They are getting used to making milk. (See Chapter 15 for more about breast care.)

Massaging milk glands

One way to help the milk flow through the milk glands in your breasts into the nipple is to massage your breasts gently with your fingertips as your baby sucks. This may help prevent ducts from getting blocked.

A blocked duct will feel like a sore lump in your breast. Massage the area and put a warm pack on it to help the milk flow through it. Let your baby nurse on that breast first.

Call the doctor or nurse if:

- A duct stays blocked for a week or more
- An area of your breast gets warm, red, and painful—signs of mastitis*

*Mastitis: An infection in the duct.

Nipple soreness

If your nipples begin to feel sore, check to make sure your baby is latching on correctly and lying with his tummy against your body. This helps keep them from getting sore. Hold your baby in different positions for feeding, so he does not always suck on your nipples the same way. Also, let your nipples dry in the air for a few minutes after each feeding.

Call quickly about breast problems

There are ways to deal with breast problems without stopping nursing. Be sure to call the nurse or breastfeeding consultant, so you can deal with the problem quickly.

Breastfeeding while working

Breastfeeding for as long as possible is best for your baby. It also helps your body recover from pregnancy. Try to keep it up for a year or more.

Many women are able to continue breastfeeding after they go back to work outside their home. Nursing when you get home is a wonderful way to feel close with your baby after being away.

You can rent or borrow an electric pump and use it at work. Pumping may seem strange at first, but it will produce a lot of milk quickly. Store the milk in a cooler. Take it home for use the next day or freeze it for next week. You can nurse your baby before leaving in the morning and in the evening. (You also can call the

A breast pump looks odd but works well.

"My three-month-old didn't want to take a bottle. My mom and I decided to try offering a bottle when he woke up from a nap."

"She held him while he slept, keeping a bottle of breast milk next to her chair. When he began to stir, she popped the nipple into his mouth and he began to suck. After that, he took one bottle happily every night."

breastfeeding consultant or La Leche League for advice about nursing when you go back to work.)

Giving a bottle if you are breastfeeding

Many breastfeeding moms want their baby to learn to take a bottle. This allows mom to be away from home for more than an hour or two. It is a good way to get a baby ready for mom's return to work. (See bottle feeding tips below.)

It is best to wait until your baby is nursing well (4 to 6 weeks). Then start offering breast milk in one bottle daily. Use a newborn nipple that has a slow flow, which is most like the breast.

Your baby may learn to take a bottle easier from your partner, a friend, or a grandparent than from you. If he is not interested in the bottle, try giving it to him just as he is waking up. This will help him understand that a bottle is just another way to get his favorite food, your milk.

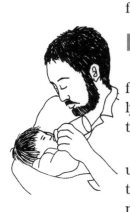

Feeding with a bottle

Whether you are using a bottle for breast milk or formula, make feeding time special. Hold your baby lying against your body with his head higher than his tummy. Look at him and talk softly.

It is very important to hold your baby. Do not prop up the bottle and leave him alone. Your baby needs the feeling of closeness he gets during feeding. He needs this time with you or other caregivers. Also, he could choke if left alone with a bottle.

Whether you are feeding breast milk or formula, be sure to:

1. Use a fresh bottle for each feeding. Do not keep unused breast milk or formula to finish later. Germs can get into the bottle and grow in the formula, even if you keep it cold.

2. Warm the bottle in a bowl of hot water for a few minutes.

Never heat a bottle in a microwave oven. The formula may get hot enough to burn your baby's mouth even if the bottle does not feel hot.

3. Test the milk by dripping a little onto the inside of your wrist. It should feel as warm as your skin.

Warming a bottle

4. Touch your baby's cheek with the nipple so he opens his mouth. Put the nipple straight in. Tip the bottle so formula fills the nipple.

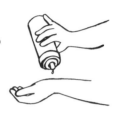

5. Stop when he shows you he has had enough. Do not push him to take more. You may be tempted to do this, because you can tell exactly how much he has taken from the bottle. Remember that each baby's appetite is different and changes often.

Testing the temperature of milk

6. Wash the bottles and nipples in hot, soapy water after every use. Nipples should be boiled before they are used for the first time.

Things to know about nipples

- Nipples come in different shapes. Your baby may like one kind better than others.

- Make sure the nipple does not flow too fast. Use a newborn-type nipple with a small hole at first. The milk should come out slowly (see pictures). If your baby starts to cough or choke, the nipple hole is probably too big.

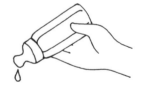

Newborn nipple with slow flow

Feeding your baby with formula

You will need to stop your breasts from making milk. See Chapter 15 for the best ways to stop your breasts from making milk.

Read the section above on bottle feeding.

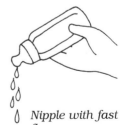

Choosing a formula

- Use only a baby formula. Cow's milk, soy, rice, or condensed milk do not have the right nutrients for a baby. Formula is made to be as much like breast milk as it can be. (However, it cannot be made with all the nourishing things in breast milk.)

Nipple with fast flow

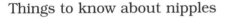

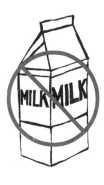

- Most babies do well on a formula based on cow's milk. If not, talk with your doctor before trying another kind. Soy-based formula is available.

- Choose formula with iron unless your baby's health care provider tells you not to do so.

- Powdered formula is the least expensive kind. It also is easiest, because you can mix it with warm water when you are ready to feed your baby.

Using formula

- To mix formula, follow the directions on the package. Be sure to measure correctly. If you use too little water or too much water, it could affect your baby's health.

- While your baby is a newborn, put only a few ounces in the bottle at one time. Always throw out any formula that he does not drink.

- Do not push your baby to take more formula than he wants. Generally, a baby under two months of age will want 2 to 4 ounces of formula every 3 to 4 hours.

- If you mix the bottles of formula ahead of time, keep them in the refrigerator. Do not let them sit at room temperature. Germs could grow in them if they are not kept cold.

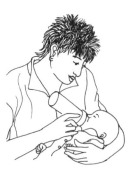

- **Warning about unclean water:** If your water comes from a well or other private source, it may not be clean enough for a newborn. If you are not sure how clean the water is, use bottled water or water that has been boiled and cooled.

  Water from pipes in old buildings may have lead in it. This is very unhealthy for babies. (See Chapter 3, under Household Hazards.)

Your baby can grow up happy and healthy with a bottle, if formula feeding is necessary.

Chapter 13

Getting to know your baby

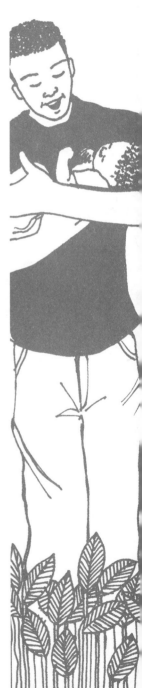

A newborn baby can do amazing things. Your baby can see your face when you hold her close and look at her. She can hear your voice. She can suck on your breast, your clean finger, or a nipple. She can hold your finger in her hand.

Until now, your baby lived curled up in a warm, dark, watery place. She heard the gurgles of your body and thumps of your heart. Now she is in the world of bright lights, sharp sounds, cool drafts, and open space. At first, loud noises make her startle or jump. Bright lights make her blink. She feels cold when she is undressed.

This chapter includes:
- Fathers and older children

Understanding your baby, page 180
- Baby's personality

How your baby develops, page 182
- Playing and talking with your baby
- Milestones of development

Sleep and crying, page 186
- Helping baby sleep
- Crying and how to deal with it

However, babies start learning about the world right away. Their brains grow and learn faster in the first three years than at any other time.

The most important people in your baby's world are you and others who care for her. Your whole family will grow together by caring for this new baby.

A good start for the whole family

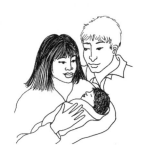

A baby grows best in a happy home. Everyone will thrive if each partner tries to understand and help each other. Mom needs help to gain strength and pay attention to the baby during the early weeks. Older children also need extra attention and love at this time.

Beginning to be a mother

Your main jobs now as a mother are to get to know your baby, feed her, and recover from delivery. (For more about your own recovery, see Chapter 15.)

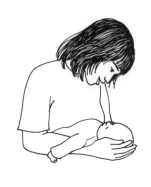

Give your baby plenty of time to suck to build up your milk supply. Nurse her in a quiet place. Play some quiet music, sip a glass of water, and relax. Make sure you are holding her in a comfortable position.

Take naps when your baby sleeps. Ask your partner and friends to do other chores, such as cooking, shopping, and laundry. If you are tired from too many visitors, it is okay to say "no." Ask them to come back in a few weeks to see the baby.

Remember that it is okay not to know exactly how to care for your baby. There are nurses and others who can give you advice or show you how to do things. Do not feel shy about calling them with questions or when you feel unsure. You will learn as you go along.

Fathering a new baby

As a father, you are very important in your baby's life. You will have your own special way of caring for your child. You will learn as you spend time with your baby.

Take time to touch, cuddle, and talk with your newborn baby. She will learn quickly to know your voice, smell, and touch. Hold her close and talk to her quietly in a singsong voice. Try caring for your baby all by yourself. Learn to diaper and bathe her, not just play with her.

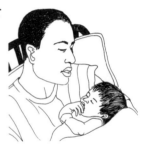

There will be a lot of work to do around the house. You will get tired during this period, too. You deserve to take some time to rest, too.

Notice how your partner is feeling. Depression* is quite common in new mothers. Watch for signs of depression, such as:

*Depression: Emotional problems after childbirth, also called Postpartum Depression.

- No appetite

- Difficulty sleeping or sleeping all the time

- No interest in caring for the baby

- Fears about her ability to take care of the baby

Some tiredness and worry are normal. However, if these emotional changes last more than two weeks, urge your partner to call your doctor or nurse-midwife right away. She may find it very hard to make the call herself.

Depression can be serious but can be treated. It is important to deal with it early. When a mom is depressed she cannot give her baby and other family members the attention and love that they need.

Older children at home

If you have other children, they may not find your new baby as exciting as you do. The baby will take most of your attention. Older children may have some behavior problems for a while. Here are some ways to help them:

- Spend some special time with each older child every day. Let them know you still love them just as much as before. You could ask close friends or family members to take the children out for some fun.

- Let older children help you with baby care, but stay with them at all times. They may not understand that they could harm your baby. For example, a 3-year-old may be eager to carry the baby but might drop her.

Warning: Do not leave the baby alone with a child under age 11 or 12. A child should not be given so much responsibility!

Other family members

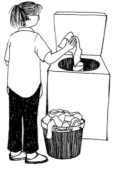

Connections with grandparents, aunts, uncles, and cousins help children grow up secure and happy. If they live nearby or are able to visit, encourage them to take part. Family members can be a big help if they are willing and able to do things around the house or with the older children.

Ask friends and relatives to help around the house.

Grandparents and other older adults may have outdated ideas of how to care for a baby. You may not agree with them. They may not understand some new ideas, such as why babies should sleep on their back or ride in a car seat. However, you should expect them to learn and follow the decisions you have made about your baby's care.

Remember that you and your partner are the parents and you make the decisions about your baby. You have tried to learn and use the best information you have found. Offer this book to your relatives. It can help them learn why you care for your baby as you do.

Help with twins, triplets, or more

If you have had twins or triplets, you and your partner certainly will need as much help as you can get. Look in Chapter 16 in this book for Mothers of Twins groups and other resources. Local support groups can give you very useful advice.

Understanding your new baby

Your newborn baby can't talk, but she does try to let you know what she wants. You, your partner, and other caretakers will learn by watching your new baby's face and body. This will help you to respect his needs.

Kinds of behavior you will see:

- **When your baby is sleepy,** her eyes will blink slowly. She will move her arms and legs more slowly and make quiet noises. She may startle more easily, especially at loud sounds. This is time to put her to bed.

- **When she is in a deep sleep,** she breathes evenly and does not wake up easily. Sometimes she will sleep more lightly. Her breathing will be less regular and her eyes may move under their lids. She may make sucking motions with her mouth and move her arms and legs.

- **When your baby is waking up** she may not be ready to eat or play. If she has been sleeping only a short time, wait a few minutes to see if she goes back to sleep. If you want to help her to wake up, talk quietly to her, rub her body, and change her diaper.

- **When she is awake and alert** she will look at you and listen to your voice. A newborn baby may only be able to do this for a minute or two at a time. When she looks away or turns her head, that is a sign that she needs to stop. Then you can simply hold her.

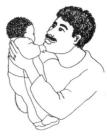

- **If your baby is fussy,** she may need your help to relax. Hold her close and rock her gently or walk with her.

- **When she is hungry,** she will suck on her fingers, turn her head toward your breast, and make soft sounds. She will cry only when she is very hungry. Try not to wait until she cries before feeding her.

"When my baby was fussy, I tried playing with her to make her feel better. It only made her cry more. I finally learned that what she needed was quiet cuddling, not more playing."

A baby's personality

Each baby shows signs of his or her own personality from the beginning. Some are very calm and quiet, watching what is going on around them. Others may be shy. Some are very active and excitable. Watch your baby to see what she is like.

How your baby develops

Your baby is born ready to play and learn, especially when you pay attention to her. Every time you hold her, talk to her, comfort her, and help her try new things, you nurture her. She feels secure when you take care of her, keep her warm and fed, and answer her cries. Feeling secure helps her brain and body develop (learn and grow) as much as possible. Babies who are not held and comforted often do not develop as well as others.

Your baby's body will grow and change every day. By six months of age, she probably will weigh twice as much as at birth. Her brain is growing very fast, so you will see her learning new things week by week.

Talking to your new baby

Your baby's brain takes in the sounds she hears from the very beginning. She is getting ready to talk and think long before she understands words. It is important for her to hear your voice and watch your face while you talk to her.

Babies love high sing-song voices. Talking slowly in a high voice helps her hear sounds clearly. You do not have to use simple "baby talk." You can look at a picture book and tell her about the pictures. Or just talk about the things you are doing. Soon she will

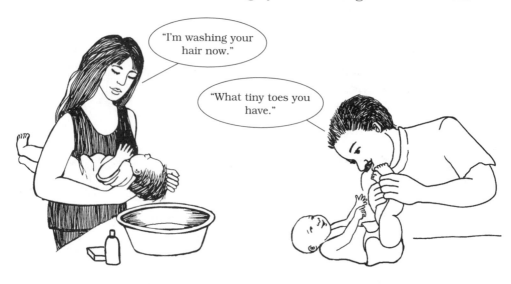

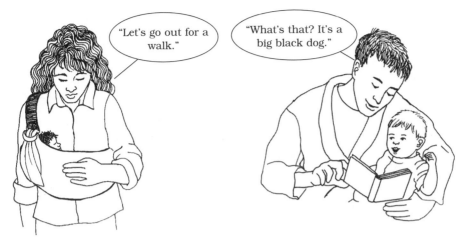

"Let's go out for a walk."

"What's that? It's a big black dog."

begin making sounds herself ("coo" and later "da-da-da"). When she does this, it is good to repeat her sounds back to her.

A baby can hear the sounds of all languages in the first six to nine months. When they get older they hear only the sounds of the language parents use with them. If you or others in your family speak other languages, it is good for your baby to hear those sounds.

Playing with your new baby

Playing helps your new baby connect with you and learn. Try these things when she is alert.

- Hold her 8 to 10 inches from your face. Smile, stick out your tongue, or make a silly face. Watch how she responds.

- Lift her gently into the air while looking at her.

- Talk to her in a high sing-song voice.

- Repeat the sounds she makes.

- Sing simple nursery songs like "Twinkle, Twinkle Little Star." Repeat the same songs often, so she will begin to know them. She will not care if you sing out-of-tune.

- Touch her gently. Stroke her arms, legs, head, and belly. Massage her body.

- Shake a rattle or a small bell. She will be interested in these sounds. Let her look at small, colorful toys that move. Soon she will want to touch and hold these things.

If your baby is a premie, she may not be very interested in playing until she gets past her original due date. She still needs to see your face, hear your voice, and feel your hands and arms holding her.

Tummy time

It is important for a baby, even a newborn, to have some time on her tummy every day. Play with her for a few minutes on her tummy two or three times daily. This gives her time to practice lifting and moving her head. Soon she will start turning it from side to side.

Lay her on a clean cloth on the floor. Place her head first to one side and then to the other. Get down beside her, so she can see your face and hands. Show her small, colorful toys. Talk to her and pat her back.

Preventing a flat spot

Some babies get flat areas on the back of their heads. This can happen if they spend a lot of time on their back in bed or in a baby seat or swing. Here are some ways to prevent a flat spot:

- When your baby is awake, give her time to lie on her tummy. You can prop her on her side to play.

- Carry her in a sling or front carrier part of the time. Hold her when she is awake.

- Make sure she does not always sleep with her head turned to the same side. Change her sleeping position so her head is at a different end of her crib each night.

- If you put her in a baby seat or swings, do it only for very short periods (See below). Use the car seat only for travel, not as a place to sleep at home.

If you think your baby might be getting a flat spot, point it out to your baby's doctor at the next checkup. Flat spots can be fixed.

Wait before using a baby seat

Wait until your baby is a few months old before using a baby seat or swing. A new baby is too young to spend much time sitting in a reclining baby seat. New babies need to lie flat most of the time or be held. Their backs and necks are not strong. During the first months, put your baby in a car seat only for car rides.

Always play gently—Never shake a baby

Make sure that anyone who plays with your baby always is very gentle. New babies have very large, heavy heads and their necks are weak. Rough play, such as bouncing a baby up and down or tossing her into the air, could injure her brain seriously. Wait until your child is much older and wants to play actively. Never, never shake your baby if you are upset.

Holding your baby

You can't spoil a new baby, so pick her up and hold her as much as you can. She needs this time in the arms of you or other caregivers. Carrying her in a sling or chest pack can help her feel comforted while you are being active.

Delays in development

Every baby develops in her own time, but each baby should make progress. Check the milestones on the next page.

Pay attention to your baby's changes. Does she show you that she can see and hear? If you have any concern about how well she is developing, tell the doctor or nurse. He may suggest waiting a while before doing anything. If so, keep close track of any changes.

If you still have concerns in a month or two, be sure to let the doctor know or talk with another health care provider. You know your baby best. The earlier your baby gets help, the more can be done to help her.

Milestones of Development

Most newborns can:

- Look at a face nearby
- Follow your face when you move side to side
- Respond to sounds (by blinking, startling, crying)
- Move arms and legs

At 1 month, most babies can:

- Respond to parent's face and voice
- Lift head briefly while lying on tummy
- Put fist in mouth
- Stop crying if picked up and cuddled

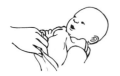

1 month

At 2 months, most babies can:

- Smile when parent smiles at her
- Look at nearby people and things
- Make soft cooing sounds at people
- Lift head, neck, and chest while lying on tummy
- Start to hold up her head when upright

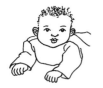

2 months

At 6 months, most babies can:

- Roll over from front to back
- Hold a small toy in her hand
- Smile, laugh, and babble
- Play with toes

If you think your baby's development is delayed, talk with the doctor.

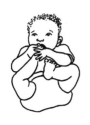

6 months

Baby's Sleep

Many newborn infants sleep most of the time and are awake for short periods. Your newborn will have periods of deep, quiet sleep and of lighter sleep. Her breathing will be fast at times and slow at other times. This is normal.

It is tempting to let your baby fall asleep while she is nursing. However, she may get in the habit of falling asleep in your arms or at the breast. It can be a difficult habit to change as she gets older.

Your baby will let you know when she needs to sleep. She will look away from you, and stop being interested in play. Her eyes will start to blink. She will yawn, rub her eyes, and make fussy noises. These are signals to put her gently into her crib on her back. She may cry briefly, but this will not harm her.

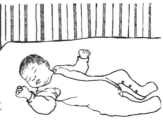

When your baby cries

Many babies have a fussy time every day during the first few months. Crying is a natural way for your baby to ask for help. It may mean she is hungry, tired, wet, lonely, uncomfortable, or sick. You will learn to know her different cries.

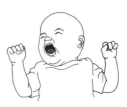

Ways to comfort a crying baby:

- First, make sure your baby is not hungry or does not have a fever or signs of illness (Chapter 15).

- Change her diaper.

- Try feeding your baby if she has not fed for an hour or more. If she is not hungry, let her suck on your clean finger or on a pacifier.

- Swaddle her snugly in a blanket.

- Hold her on her tummy and rock her.

- Put your baby in a sling, or front pack and walk with her in the house or outside.

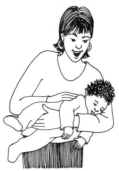

Babies like to be held with mom's hand against their tummy.

- Try repeating sounds in her ear, like "shhh, shhh, shhh," over and over again. Some babies like the sound of the clothes dryer.

- If she has been awake for a long time, she may be very tired. She may need to cry for a few minutes in her crib before she can sleep.

If your baby cries often and you can't soothe her, talk with her doctor or nurse practitioner to make sure there is no medical cause. Some foods may bother her or she may have reflux.*

*Reflux: Gastroesophageal reflux, a painful condition caused by acid from the stomach backing up into the esophagus. There are ways to treat reflux in babies.

Colic

Some babies have colic, times when they cry hard for hours at a time. The crying remedies above may not help. There is not treatment, but colic does not harm the baby. She will outgrow it by 3 or 4 months of age.

Parents usually get very upset because they are not able to comfort their baby. This is one of the hardest things you may face. Talking with a friend may help you deal with your frustration. Try to get some exercise and enough sleep.

If you find yourself getting angry with your baby, put her in her crib while you calm down. Remind yourself that she is not doing this to make you upset. Avoid taking alcohol or drugs when you are feeling this way.

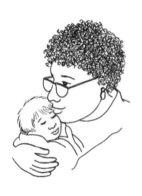

Find a friend or relative you trust to babysit, so you can have an hour or two away. Leave your baby only with a person who you know will be able to handle the crying without becoming very upset. Some adults can't handle it and might harm a crying baby.

NEVER shake your baby to try to make her stop crying. First, it will not work. Second, shaking can injure her brain very seriously.

Chapter 14

Keeping Your Baby Safe

The biggest dangers to healthy babies during the first few months are from SIDS (Sudden Infant Death Syndrome) and car crashes. SIDS rarely affects babies after the first year. Car crashes, however, kill or hurt children of all ages.

It is hard to imagine that sleeping or riding in a car could hurt your baby. They are things we all do every day. Most of the time, nothing harmful happens. Yet, every parent—and every other caregiver—needs to pay attention to keeping babies safe.

Neither SIDS nor car-crash injury can be prevented completely. However, there are things you can do to greatly lessen the chance of death or injury.

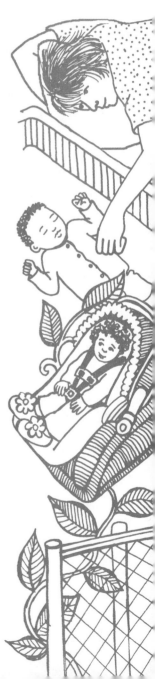

This chapter includes:

Sleep safety—Preventing SIDS, page 190

- Many helpful things to do
- Safe places to sleep

Car seat safety, page 193

- Buckling baby into a car seat
- Installing the seat in the car
- Practical tips

Other safety concerns, page 196

- Preventing falls and burns
- Baby-proofing your home

Sleep Safety

Preventing SIDS*

SIDS: Sudden Infant Death Syndrome, sometimes called "crib death."

SIDS is the death of a baby under age 1 that cannot be medically explained. It usually happens when the baby is sleeping. It is most likely between age 1 month and 6 months.

No one knows how to prevent it completely. No one can be blamed if a baby dies of SIDS. However, there are a number of simple things that have been found to lower the chance of sudden infant death.

Always put your baby to sleep on his back.

The safest position for a healthy baby is on his back. Babies who sleep that way from birth generally like it. Side-sleeping is less safe than back-sleeping.

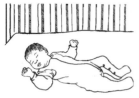

Some parents fear that a baby sleeping on his back could spit up and choke. This has not been found to be true for healthy babies.

Premature infants who have needed to sleep on their tummies in the hospital should be switched to back-sleeping before going home. Find out from the doctor if there is a medical reason for your baby to continue sleeping on his tummy.

By the time a baby learns to roll over, the risk of SIDS is less than before. Continue to put him to bed on his back.

Other important ways to help prevent SIDS

- Put your baby on his back in a crib with a very firm mattress.
- Put no blankets over him.
- Dress him in pajamas that will keep him warm but not hot without a blanket. Keep the room a comfortable temperature for you. If he wakes up sweaty or with a red face he has been too hot.
- Put no soft blankets, pillows, quilts, sheepskins, and stuffed toys in your baby's crib. These can cover his face and limit his breathing as he moves during sleep. (Put these things away until his first birthday.)

- Keep your baby's bed in the room where you sleep. However, sharing the same bed can be risky (see next page).

- Give your baby a pacifier when he goes to sleep. For breastfed babies, wait until breastfeeding is going well (usually about one month) before starting a pacifier. (Offer the pacifier for sleep even if your baby does not want it when awake.)

- Breastfeed your baby.

- Do not smoke in your home or car, especially around your baby. Ask others who smoke to do so outside.

- Keep your baby away from crowds and people with colds.

NOTE: Make sure everyone who cares for your baby **always** puts him to sleep on his back. Tell grandparents and child care providers why this is important. When a baby is used to sleeping on his back, SIDS can happen if he is mistakenly put to sleep on his tummy just once.

A safe sleeping place for a baby

Your baby's crib should meet current safety standards (see Chapter 6) and should have a firm, tightly fitting mattress.

SIDS danger is higher for babies sleeping:

- In a bed with an adult or child

- On a soft sofa, couch, or waterbed

- With an adult who has been using alcohol or drugs (an adult sleeping very soundly who could roll onto the baby)

Sharing a bed

Many parents like to have their baby sleep in their room or in their bed. However, new research shows that bed-sharing can increase the chance of SIDS.

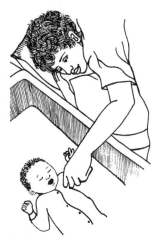

Baby's crib next to parents' bed

The safest way to have your baby near you is to put the crib or basket next to the bed. If he falls asleep in your bed, you can move him to the crib easily.

If you are determined to have your baby sleep in your bed, pay special attention to making the bed safe. Make sure:

- There are no pillows and heavy blankets or quilts over or near the baby.

- The mattress is very firm.

- There is no gap between the bed and the wall or headboard, where the baby's head could get stuck.

- There is no way for the baby to roll off the edge of the bed.

- The baby does not sleep between two adults.

Preventing a flattened head

The back of some babies' heads may get flatter in the early months. A baby's head is growing and can change shape easily. It is most likely to get flat if a baby spends a lot of time lying on his back or sitting in a baby seat or car seat when awake.

Ways to prevent flattening:

- Make sure your baby has plenty of time lying on his tummy or in your arms while he is awake.

- Avoid sitting him in a baby seat or swing for long periods. Use a car seat only for travel.

- Change the position of his head when he is lying on his back. Tilt his head to one side or the other. Put his head toward one end of the crib for one night and the other end for the next night.

Watch the shape of your baby's head. If you think it is changing, show his doctor right away. Follow the suggestions above. There are ways to re-shape his head if necessary.

Buckling up baby on every ride

A car safety seat can save a child's life. But it can only work if it is used on every trip. It also must be the right size and be used correctly.

If you do not have a car seat yet, see Chapter 6 for details on how to choose one.

Follow the instructions that came with the car seat. Also read "About child restraints" in the vehicle owner's manual.

Remember to always buckle up yourself. Your baby needs you to be safe so you can care for him.

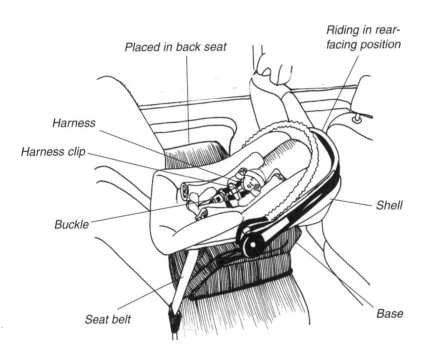

Features of car safety seats

Installing the seat in the car

Put the car seat in the back seat facing the rear. The back seat has been proven to be much safer than the front for children up to at least age 13.   The rear-facing position is safest because it cushions the baby's head, neck, and back inside the shell.

Use the center of the back seat if the car seat can be installed tightly there and you are not carrying other children. However, in some cars the vehicle seat has a hump so a car seat does not fit there.

Recline the car seat just enough so your baby's head does not fall forward. It should not be reclined more than half-way back. Many car seats have a recline indicator. Most infant-only seats have a recline adjuster, too. If the car seat does not have one, wedge a rolled towel or foam "pool noodle" under the car seat below the baby's feet to tilt it back slightly.

Install the car seat tightly with either a safety belt or the new LATCH* system. Check your vehicle owner's manual to learn how to use these systems. The seat should move no more than one inch side to side and forward when installed.

*LATCH: A new way of securing a car seat in a vehicle with special hardware in newer vehicles and car seats.

- Decide first where you want your baby to ride. If you want to put him in the middle of the back seat, you may need to use the seat belt. Few vehicles have LATCH anchors there.

- There are several kinds of belts that are tightened around a car seat in different ways.

- To use the LATCH system, both the vehicle and the car seat must have special parts that connect together. Often, but not always, LATCH provides a tighter installation than the seat belt. If not, use the seat belt.

If your baby must ride in front

Never place your baby in the front seat with an air bag unless it has been turned off. Front passenger air bags can be deadly to rear-facing infants. Put the car seat in front only if there is no place for it in the back seat.

If a sports car or pickup truck has no back seat, or a very small one, the vehicle will either have sensors or an on-off switch for the air bag. If it has a switch, you must remember to turn off the air bag while a baby or child is riding in front. (Turn it on again when adults and teens are seated there.)

More and more new vehicles have sensors that automatically shut off the air bag if a small child is buckled into the front seat. Read the owner's manual. Check the indicator light in the dashboard to make sure the air bag is off when your baby rides in front.

If you have an older car and are not sure it has a front passenger air bag, check for a label on the sun visor or read the owner's manual.

Buckling your new baby in the car seat

- The crotch strap must go between his legs.
- Shoulder straps must go over his shoulders. The straps should come from the seat as close as possible to the shoulders or slightly below them.
- The harness must be snug. To test it, pinch the strap between your fingers (see picture). If you can pinch any slack, it is not snug enough.
- Put the harness clip at the level of your baby's armpits.

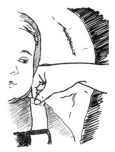

Pinch the strap to see if it is too loose.

Practical car seat tips

- Pad the sides of the car seat to keep your newborn from slumping. Some car seats come with padded inserts. If not, put rolled blankets or diapers along both sides of your baby's body and head. Do not put padding under him.

  Avoid using a head-support pad you can purchase separately. It might allow the baby to be thrown out in a crash.

- Dress your baby in clothes with legs. The harness straps must go between his legs. Never wrap your baby in a blanket before putting him into the car seat.

- If the weather is cold, put your baby in a fleece sleeper with legs. Do not use a bulky snowsuit. Tuck a blanket over the straps.

Getting help with car seat use

Car seats can be confusing to use correctly. You may want to have your car seat checked by a certified

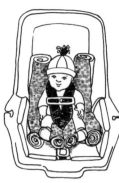

Pad the sides of the car seat with rolled receiving blankets.

Child Passenger Safety Technician near you. Locate a technician or a car seat inspection site through the SeatCheck web site or phone line (see Chapter 17).

Car bed for special needs

A rear-facing car seat is best, but some babies may have a medical need to lie flat. There are a few car beds made for babies who must lie flat (see SafetyBeltSafe, U.S.A. listing, Chapter 17).

Premature babies born earlier than 37 weeks should be testing sitting in their car seat before leaving the hospital, according to the American Academy of Pediatrics. If the baby shows signs of breathing problems, the baby should travel lying flat. (He also should not sit in a swing or baby seat at home until he is older.) If your baby is a premie, ask your baby's doctor or nurse about "apnea testing" in a car seat.

Keep your baby safe from falls

A baby needs safe places, such as:

- A crib with slats close together will keep him from slipping through.

- A changing table with sides will help keep him from rolling off.

- A clean space on the floor for play. Lay him on a clean blanket on his tummy. When he begins to crawl, be sure to put gates on the stairs.

When you change, bathe, or dress your baby, **keep one hand on his body so he doesn't fall.** Have everything you need within reach before you start.

Preventing burns, scalds, and fire

Your baby's skin is very thin and can be easily burned or scalded. Ways to prevent burns:

- **Scalding:** Do not hold a hot drink while your baby is in your arms. Drink your coffee while he is playing on the floor or sleeping.

- Make sure the bath water is no hotter than lukewarm. Test it with your elbow. Turn down the temperature of your hot water heater to 120 degrees.

- **Heaters:** When your baby starts to crawl, put gates or fences up around the fireplace, wood stove, and electric heaters.

- **Sunburn:** When your baby is outside in the middle of the day (10 AM to 4 PM), keep him in the shade or dress him in light clothes that cover his arms and legs. After 6 months of age, use sunscreen made for children. Keeping him out of the sun is the best protection.

Check your home smoke alarms

Smoke detectors can save your whole family from a house fire. Make sure your home has at least one detector on each level, especially outside bedroom doors.

Change the batteries at least once a year. Pick a date you will remember, like your baby's birthday, for changing them. Use the test button every month, too, to make sure the alarms are working.

Baby-proofing your house

As your baby learns to crawl, walk, and climb, there will be many things to do to make your home safer. The best way to protect your baby is to keep dangerous things out of reach. Also, if things are put away, you will not have to watch your baby every minute and tell him "no" constantly.

"I could hardly believe all the tiny things my baby could find on the floor. He must have wonderful eyesight. I found I needed to sweep every day while he was crawling."

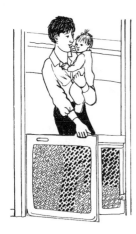

Sweep or vacuum the floor often. Crawling babies will find even the smallest piece of dust or dirt and put it in their mouths.

Put breakable or dangerous things out of reach when he shows signs of beginning to crawl.

Put gates on stairs and keep them closed.

You will need to keep checking your home for hazards during your baby's first few years of life. Make sure that other homes where your baby spends time are also baby-proofed.

Chapter 15

Keeping Your Baby Healthy

Many health and developmental problems can be prevented or lessened by good health care. Part of good health care is taking your baby for regular checkups. Getting your child immunized on time also is very important. You also need to know the signs of illness, when to call the doctor or nurse, and the basic kinds of home care your sick baby might need.

Keys to your baby's health

- Breastfeed your baby to give her some of your antibodies to fight germs.

- Wash your hands often during the day and make sure others do, too.

- Take your baby for regular checkups.

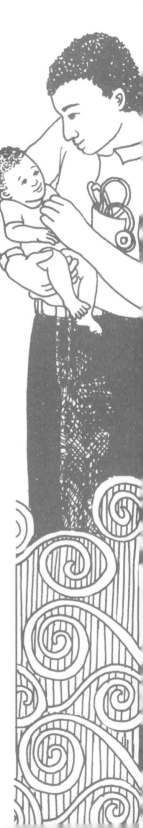

This chapter includes:

Basics of keeping your baby healthy, page 199

- Hand washing

- Well-baby checkups

Immunizations, page 202

- Vaccines

- Immunization schedule

Signs of illness, page 207

- Care when your baby is sick

- Keep her away from people who are smoking. Ask visitors and family members who smoke to do it outside.

- Keep your baby away from people who have colds, coughs, or other illnesses that spread easily. They may not seem very sick but could still spread illnesses that are serious for babies.

- Avoid taking her into crowded places, like malls and movie theaters, for the first few months.

- Make sure your baby gets her immunizations (shots) on time to prevent serious illnesses.

Hand washing

Make sure everyone who cares for your baby washes his or her hands. This simple task is the best way to prevent the spread of common germs.

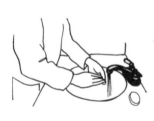

- Wash your hands **before** handling or playing with your baby and before preparing food.

- Wash them **after** using the bathroom, changing her diaper, handling raw foods, or blowing your nose.

- Wash hands more often if you have a cold or other illness. (If you are coughing, do not use your hand to cover your mouth. Instead, turn your head and cough into your sleeve.)

- Wash after going out to the store.

- Make sure older children wash after returning from child care or school or from playing outside. They should not touch the baby if they have colds.

Hand sanitizers and anti-bacterial soaps

Avoid using anti-bacterial cleaning products on your hands or in your home. They can harm long-term health by making bacteria resistant to antibiotic drugs. That means those drugs will not work well against serious infections in the future.

A hand sanitizer (cleaner) made with alcohol can help prevent the spread of viruses like colds. This kind of cleaner does not make bacteria resistant.

How to wash your hands well

1) Use warm water and soap or a "hand sanitizer." It is not helpful to use anti-bacterial soap. Most common illnesses, such as colds, are caused by viruses, not bacteria.

2) Rub soapy hands together for 15 to 20 seconds (the time it takes to hum the "Happy Birthday" song slowly). It can take that long to really get the germs out of finger nails and creases.

3) Rinse and dry with a clean towel.

Your baby's checkups

Health tests after birth

Your new baby will have a number of tests done in the hospital or birth center. These include overall health, hearing, and development. (Many newborns are given their first immunization for Hepatitis B at the hospital.)

A nurse will take a tiny bit of blood from your baby's heel to test (screen) for a number of rare but very serious diseases. Any such disease that is found and treated right away can save a baby from serious, lifelong health problems.

In many states, all babies are required to have the blood test repeated 7 to 14 days after birth. **If your provider asks you to bring your baby in for a second test, it is important to do so.** The second test may find problems that did not show up right after birth.

Well-baby checkups

Your baby's doctor will want to check her within the first week. Your baby should have regular checkups five or six times during the first year.

Why does a healthy baby need to visit the doctor?

The doctor or nurse practitioner can learn whether your baby is growing normally by checking her body, growth, and development. He may find problems that you cannot see. Finding such problems early can keep

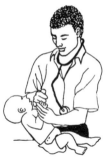

them from becoming serious. Your baby also will get immunizations at checkups. The checkup is a good chance to ask questions about your baby's care and development.

What happens at a well-baby checkup?

At each checkup, the doctor or nurse will weigh your baby and measure her length and head size. He will check her ears, eyes, mouth, lungs, heart, abdomen, genitals, hips, legs, and reflexes.

He will check your baby's development. He will look for the things she is learning to do, such as holding up her head and smiling. Be sure to tell him the new things that you have seen your baby do.

Asking questions

The checkup is the best time to ask the doctor or nurse any questions you have. (When you visit the doctor with a sick baby, you may not have time to talk about other concerns.) But, it may be hard to remember all the things you want to talk about. Write down your questions when you think of them at home. Take the list to the next checkup.

It also helps to write down the answers when you talk with your baby's health care provider. This will help you remember exactly what he said.

Baby's immunization record

Use the record page at the end of this chapter to keep track of your baby's early checkups and immunizations.

Your clinic or health department will give you a card to keep a list of your baby's checkups and immunizations. You will need this information if you change doctors or move to another town. Keep this card in a safe place and bring it to all your baby's checkups.

Immunizations are lifesavers

Why do babies need immunizations?

Your baby should be immunized to protect (immunize) her from some very serious diseases that spread easily from person to person. Before immunizations were made for diseases such as diphtheria, polio, and tetanus, many people died from those diseases or had lifelong disability.

Thanks to immunizations, many dangerous diseases are rare in this country today. Parents today may not realize how very dangerous they can be. However, outbreaks of measles and whooping cough have happened in the U.S. recently.

Outbreaks happen because some people who had not been immunized got sick. They passed germs on to babies who had not been given vaccine yet. Some babies die in outbreaks or survive with long-term health problems. Immunizing your baby helps protect her and the whole community.

A vaccine is the substance that your baby is given to make her immune. For full protection, several doses of some vaccines are needed. All states require children to have a number of immunizations before starting child care or school. Doctors advise giving several other kinds that are not required.

"I was glad to get my baby immunized. Now I don't have to worry that someone might pass a serious illness to my child,"

Get your baby fully immunized by 15 to 18 months of age

Don't wait until your child goes to school or child care. She could be harmed most by some diseases during her first few years.

Babies must get more than one dose of most vaccines to have full protection. Older children and adults also must get "booster shots" of some vaccines because protection may fade over the years. Flu vaccine is given each year because the influenza germ changes from year to year.

There are 9 vaccines made to prevent 13 diseases as of 2006. More are being developed. A vaccine to prevent rotavirus (severe diarrhea) may be added to the list very soon. In the future, vaccines may be combined so fewer injections are needed.

It may seem hard for your baby to get so many injections. Remember that the pain lasts only a few minutes but the benefit lasts for years or a lifetime. To comfort your baby, cuddle her, distract her with a favorite blanket or soft toy, or nurse her.

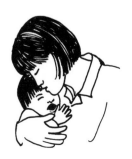

Vaccines Recommended – 2006

Vaccine	Number of doses	Age when doses are given
DTaP:	5 doses	At 2 months, 4 months, 6 months, 15–18 months, 4–6 years
Hep A	2 doses	For children over 24 months in high-risk areas only
Hep B:	3 doses	At birth, 1–4 months, 6–18 months
Hib	4 doses	At 2 months, 4 months, 6 months, 12–15 months
Influenza	Annually	At 6 months or more, given in flu season (2 doses for children getting this vaccine for the first time)
MMR	2 doses	At 12–15 months, 4–6 years
PCV	4 doses	At 2 months, 4 months, 6 months, 12–15 months
Polio (IPV)	4 doses	At 2 months, 4 months, 6–18 months, 4–6 years
Varicella	1 dose	At 12–18 months

The diseases vaccines prevent

Many of these diseases are rare today. Without vaccines, however, they would be very serious.

- **DTaP** for diphtheria, tetanus, and pertussis.

    Diphtheria (dif-thee-ree-a) can cause heart and breathing problems, paralysis, or death.

    Tetanus (lockjaw) causes severe muscle and breathing problems and, often, death.

    Pertussis (whooping cough) can cause severe coughing, lung problems, seizures, brain damage, or death in babies, but is mild in adults.

- **Hep A** for hepatitis A, a liver disease that is spread through food, water, and dirty hands.

- **Hep B** for hepatitis B, a serious liver infection that can pass from mother to baby.

- **Hib** (or HBCV) for haemophilus influenzae b (hay-ma-fill-us in-flew-en-zay b, which causes meningitis (brain swelling) and can lead to brain damage.

- **Influenza** for "the flu", the same immunization given every year to adults.

- **MMR** for measles, mumps, and rubella (German measles).

  Measles can cause deafness, brain damage, or death.

  Mumps can cause deafness, brain damage.

  Rubella (German measles) can cause brain damage in unborn babies if passed from a child to a pregnant woman.

- **PCV** for pneumococcal (new-mo-cock-al) disease, which can cause brain disease, blood infections, and pneumonia (new-mo-nee-ah).

- **Polio** (IPV) for polio, which can cause life-long paralysis or death.

- **Varicella** for chicken pox, which can cause pneumonia and brain swelling, most serious in infants and in teens and adults.

Talk with your baby's doctor or nurse if you have questions or concerns about immunizations. There is a lot of incorrect information in the news about the safety of vaccines.

Common questions about immunizations

Can immunizations be given even when my baby has a cold? Yes, getting vaccines when she has a mild illness will do no harm.

What if we miss a well-baby checkup? Make another appointment and go in soon so you can keep your baby's immunizations up-to-date.

What side effects should I expect after immunizations? Some will give your baby no side effects. After others, your baby may have redness where the shot was given. She may be fussy for a few days. Ask the doctor or nurse what to expect and the best ways to comfort your baby.

Could several injections given at one time harm a baby? No, although it can be hard for parents to watch. Each injection does hurt for a short time.

Can a baby get seriously ill from an immunization? It is very, very rare for a baby to have a severe reaction. However, if your baby seems to be sick after an immunization, be sure to call the doctor or nurse.

If I do not want my child to get a required immunization, can she still go to child care or school? A child who is not immunized can go, but parents must sign a state waiver form. If an outbreak of disease happens, the child could be required to stay away from other children.

Not being immunized is a serious public health matter. Parents must understand that a child who does not get all her immunizations could catch a serious, preventable illness from others. She also could spread that illness to others easily.

When your baby gets sick

Call the doctor or nurse if your baby is looking or behaving differently from usual. You will soon learn what is normal for her. If you are worried, it is best to talk with your health care provider. If your insurance or health plan has a consulting nurse, you also could call that number. Doctors and nurses expect new parents to call as often as necessary. The only silly questions are the ones you don't ask.

If you cannot reach your doctor or nurse after office hours, take your baby to the emergency room. If you think your baby's life could be in danger, call 9-1-1.

Warning signs: first few months

Any of these signs could mean your baby has a serious illness. Call right away if your baby has:

- **Skin that looks yellow** (jaundice), most serious in the first 24 hours after birth, but much more common in the first week after birth or in the second and third week if you are breast-feeding.

- **Infected umbilical cord or circumcised penis:** bright red blood or white pus* and a red area around the cord stump or tip of the penis.

  Pus: Gooey, smelly, white or yellow discharge from an infected wound.

- **Temperature** under about 97° F or over 100° F (when taken in the armpit) or over 100.2° (taken rectally), when not dressed too warmly. Always use a thermometer, not your hands, to decide if your baby has a fever.

- **No appetite:** no interest in breast or bottle for two feedings in a row.

- **Coughing or choking** while feeding (except if breast milk or formula is flowing too fast).

- **No wet diapers** in 12 hours (Putting a tissue inside a disposable diaper helps you know if it gets wet.)

- **Vomiting with force** (shooting 2 or 3 feet out of baby's mouth) or vomiting that goes on for more than 6 hours. (Sometimes a normal burp can seem forceful.)

- **Diarrhea** (die-a-ree-ah): two or more bowel movements that are green and watery, or more than 8 soft stools in 24 hours.

- **Tummy that feels very hard** or full.

- **Liquid or blood oozing from any opening.** (Except it is normal for a newborn girl to have a little blood or milky flow from her vagina during the first week. Also some babies' breasts ooze a little milk in the first days.)

- **Thick yellow-green mucus** in baby's nose.

- **Breathing problems**

  - Breathing too fast—more than 60 breaths per minute (babies normally breathe much faster than adults do)

  - Very heavy breathing, having a hard time breathing

  - Wheezing or grunting sounds

  - No breaths for more than 15 seconds

- **Bluish skin, lips, or tongue** (except a baby's hands and feet when they are cold, or her face when she is crying very hard).

- **More crying than usual,** especially high-pitched shrieks.

- **Sleepier than usual,** little movement, or baby's body is very floppy.

Before calling the doctor:

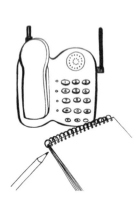

- Take your baby's temperature if you think she may have a fever. Write down how high it is, whether you took it in the armpit or rectum, and at what time.

- Make notes of the symptoms or things that concern you (for example: pale skin, sharp cry, dry stools, vomiting, or diarrhea).

- Have a pencil and paper ready when you call, so you can write down what the doctor or nurse tells you.

Call your health care provider's office or consulting nurse. The doctor or nurse will give you ideas about things you can do at home to help your baby feel better. He may ask you to bring your baby into the office or go to an urgent-care clinic or emergency room.

Some illnesses to know

Newborn Jaundice: Yellowing of the skin, caused by unusual amounts of "bilirubin" in the blood. Slight yellowing can happen because the newborn's liver is not functioning well. This may happen during the first few weeks after birth. This kind may not need treatment. The more serious kind of jaundice often starts in the first day after birth. The baby's skin, even the palms of the hands, will get very yellow. Serious jaundice can lead to brain damage if it is not treated.

RSV: A serious virus, which starts like a common cold but gets much worse rapidly. The baby may have a very hard time breathing. (It is spread by dirty hands, so hand washing is very important to keep your baby from catching it.)

Rotavirus: Severe diarrhea with vomiting and fever. It can lead to serious dehydration. (It also is spread easily by dirty hands, so be sure to wash hands often.)

Fever: Taking your baby's temperature

Fever is a sign that your baby's body is fighting an illness. You can't know your baby has a fever just by feeling her forehead. Her doctor or nurse practitioner will want to know exactly how high the fever is.

Use a digital thermometer. It is safer, easier, and faster to use than an old-fashioned glass thermometer. Practice taking your baby's temperature when she is not sick. This will give you an idea of what her normal temperature is.

There are several ways to take a baby's temperature:

- in the armpit (axillary method) gives the lowest reading, normal is 97.6° F.

- in the rectum (rectal method) gives the highest reading, normal is 99.6° F.

- in the ear (tympanic method) uses a special thermometer and is advised only after 3 months of age. It also gives a high reading.

Taking a temperature by mouth (orally) is for older children and adults. It gives a normal reading of 98.6° F.

Ask your health care provider which way she prefers. Ask how high it should be before you call. When you tell her your baby's temperature, be sure to tell which way you took it.

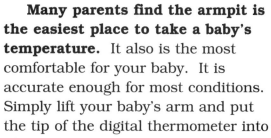

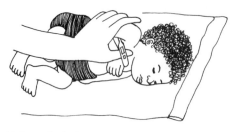

Many parents find the armpit is the easiest place to take a baby's temperature. It also is the most comfortable for your baby. It is accurate enough for most conditions. Simply lift your baby's arm and put the tip of the digital thermometer into her armpit. Then lower her arm and hold it down against her body. The digital thermometer beeps when it is done.

Taking baby's temperature in the armpit

Giving medicine to a baby

It is easiest to give a baby liquid medicine. A medicine syringe or special spoon makes it easy to put the medicine in the baby's mouth. A syringe is best for measuring and giving small amounts of medicine. (You can get these at a drug store.)

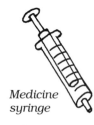

Medicine syringe

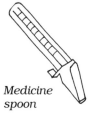

Medicine spoon

Make sure you give the right amount of medicine. This usually depends on the child's weight and age. For example, under 6 months of age, Tylenol should be given only if your baby's doctor tells you it is okay. He would tell you how much to give. For older babies, check the dosage listed on the package.

Giving antibiotics

If the doctor has prescribed an antibiotic drug, make sure to give the drug for the full length of time. Stopping it too soon may make it work less well the next time your baby needs it.

Antibiotic drugs work only with illnesses caused by bacteria, such as strep throat. They do not cure illnesses caused by viruses, such as colds. Using an antibiotic when it is **not** needed can be harmful. It makes germs stronger, so the drugs will not work when they are needed in the future.

This is also true about antibiotic soaps sold for home use. These can do more harm than good and should not be used.

Using the emergency room

Take your baby to the emergency room only in a real emergency, like a sudden, serious injury or serious illness.

In most cases, your baby's regular doctor or nurse practitioner can give her the best care when she is sick. Try to call the health care provider first. He or another doctor or nurse who works with him should be available to talk with you, even at night, and to tell you the best place to go for treatment.

Keep track of your baby's checkups and immunizations on the next page.

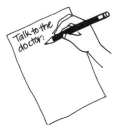

Your baby's first checkups

Newborn Screening

__ First blood screen (before going home)

__ Second blood screen (if required in your state) in the second week

Comments: _____

Well-Baby Checkups

The exact schedule will depend on your baby's health and on your health care provider or insurance plan.

First checkup (1–2 weeks)   (date) _____

Baby's age ___ weeks; weight ___ pounds, ___ ounces;

Length ___ inches; head size ___ inches

Comments: _____

_____

_____

Date and time of next checkup: _____

Second checkup (2 months)   (date) _____

Baby's age ___ weeks; weight ___ pounds, ___ ounces;

Length ___ inches; head size ___ inches

Comments: _____

_____

_____

Date and time of next checkup (usually at 4 months): _____

First Immunizations	Dates given
Hep B: first at birth to 2 months	_____
DTP: first at 2 months	_____
Polio: first at 2 months	_____
Hib: first at 2 months	_____

Chapter 16

Taking Care of Yourself

Mom, remember to take care of your own health, too! You need to recover from delivery in order to take the best care of your baby.

During the first few weeks after birth, you need plenty of rest and time to get to know your baby. Let others do the housework.

Try to take a nap whenever your baby is sleeping. You will need the sleep! Forget all the extra things around the house you think you should do.

Getting help at home

You do not have to do all the work at home. Your partner, friends, and family will want to help you at this special time. They could do household chores like

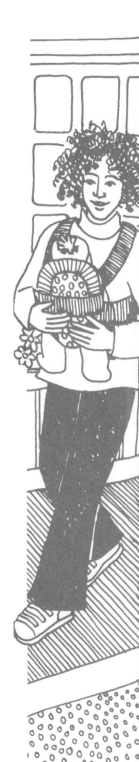

This chapter includes:

- Help at home

What to expect as your body heals, page 214

- Warning signs
- Recovery from cesarean section
- Breast care
- Eating right

Your 6-week checkup, page 218

- Family planning

Depression after childbirth, page 220

doing laundry and washing dishes. They could bring cooked foods for your family and go shopping for you. Let them do things that would take you away from your baby and his needs.

Many people will be happy to help but they may want to know what you need most. It is okay to tell them what you need help with. Be sure you do not feel you must take care of them. You do not need to entertain guests now. You also may find that you want time alone with your baby. It is okay to say "no visitors today."

One visitor you probably will welcome in the first few days is a visiting nurse. This is a wonderful service, giving you time with a skilled health care professional. She will be able to answer questions about your baby's needs and your own recovery. She can demonstrate how to do things that you are not sure about.

What to expect as your body heals

- **You will have pink or brownish discharge** from your vagina for a few weeks. Use pads only, never tampons. If you are too active, your flow may turn bright red again. If you have heavy bleeding or if the discharge smells bad, call your doctor or nurse-midwife.

- **Your uterus will get smaller rapidly.** Your weight will come down too. Use the Kegel squeeze and the pelvic tilt (page 95) to help your tummy and vagina get back in shape.

- **If you had an episiotomy or tear,** your perineum will be sore. Warm baths or Witch Hazel pads (Tucks) will be soothing. Keep the area clean. Change your pads often.

- **If you had stitches in your perineum you may worry that they will pull out** when you have a bowel movement. If so, hold some toilet paper against the stitches while you push.

- **If you have trouble urinating,** drink lots of water. Urinating in the shower or pouring warm water over your vulva while sitting on the toilet may help. If you still need help, call your doctor or nurse midwife.

- **To prevent constipation,** eat fresh fruits and vegetables, bran cereal, and prunes. Drink 8 to 10 glasses of water a day.

"I tried eating lots of fruits and veggies but I was still constipated. When I started drinking lots of water, too, it worked better. Prune juice worked really well."

Warning signs: The first few weeks

Call your doctor or nurse-midwife if you have:

- heavy bleeding—bright red blood or clots that soak your menstrual pad in an hour or less

- discharge from your vagina that smells bad

- fever

- trouble urinating or having bowel movements

- pain in the genital area or the uterus

- incision (episiotomy or cesarean) that shows signs of infection (pus, redness, soreness, or swelling)

- breasts that are painful (after your milk has come in and your breasts are less engorged); breast that have warm, red areas; nipples that are cracked or sore

- legs that are swollen or a warm, red, tender area in one leg

- problems sleeping (when baby sleeps) or feeling very emotional or sad (especially if the mood continues for two weeks or more)

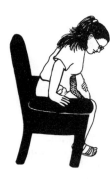

Holding a pillow over your stitches makes it less painful to get up.

Recovering after a C-section

If you had a Cesarean section, you may have a lot of pain for a while. You will need extra help with home chores such as cooking, cleaning, and the laundry. Try not to get overtired. That would slow your recovery and may give you less energy for your baby.

Sleep as much as you can but also get up and move around. Staying in bed is not healthy. Walk around the house and spend time sitting in a chair several times a day. It is likely to be painful to stand up. Hold a pillow firmly over your incision while getting up from the bed or chair.

Use your energy to breastfeed and cuddle your baby. Nursing may be most comfortable if you lie on your side or sit with your baby in the football position. Let others change your baby's diapers or walk him up and down to help him sleep.

Breast care

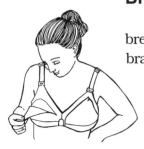

Use a strong bra that is large enough to support your breasts. You may be more comfortable wearing a nursing bra all the time, even at night.

It is not necessary to wash your nipples before or after each feeding. In fact, that can make them sore. Just let them dry in the air for a few minutes after nursing. Wash them normally when you bathe daily.

If one of your nipples feels sore, you can try putting a cool, soaked tea bag on it. Also check to make sure your baby is lying facing your breast. Make sure he is latching on properly. (See Chapter 12 for more on breast care).

Be sure to call your nurse or breastfeeding consultant right away if:

- A nipple gets cracked or starts bleeding
- A breast has a red, sore area, with fever, headache, or flu symptoms

If you are not nursing

If you have decided not to breastfeed, your breasts will need to stop making milk. This usually takes about a week. You can help this happen without using drugs. Ways to do this are:

- Wear a supportive bra and avoid touching your breasts as much as possible.
- Use a pain reliever such as Tylenol.
- Put ice packs on your breasts on the armpit side several times each day. Avoid getting hot water on your breasts when bathing or showering.
- Drink less fluid for a few days.

Keep up your healthy habits

You can help your body heal. Follow the healthy food habits you started in pregnancy (Chapter 4). You need to eat well to gain strength and energy. Eat plenty of protein and calcium from meat, fish, beans, milk, and cheese. If you are breastfeeding twins or triplets, you will need to eat more food to make larger amounts of milk.

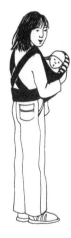

Start exercising gently again. Walking is the best way to begin. You can take your baby along in a sling or front carrier. He will enjoy the motion and being cuddled against your chest. If you had a Cesarean, ask your doctor before starting to exercise.

There are simple exercises you can do for your stomach and back. Your doctor or nurse-midwife can give you some details. Before you do more vigorous exercise, check with your health care provider.

Remember how to lift safely as you begin to carry and lift your baby. Keep a straight back and bend your knees when picking him up.

Avoid alcohol and other drugs

Being a new mother can be hard, but alcohol, cigarettes, and other drugs can make it harder. All of these things damage your health. They can also make it harder—not easier—for you to handle the difficult parts of parenting.

If you are breastfeeding, these drugs might harm your baby's brain and growth. Breast milk carries alcohol, nicotine, and other drugs to your baby.

Smoke in the air your baby breathes can give him health problems, too. Babies of smokers generally have more colds, ear infections, and a higher risk of SIDS. Anyone who smokes should do so outside the house and not in the car.

Your own six-week checkup

You should see your doctor or nurse-midwife at least once about six weeks after delivery. He will want to check how your body is recovering, how you are feeling, and help you decide what kind of birth control may be best for you.

You do not need to wait until this visit if you have urgent questions. Call your health care provider any time.

Thinking about birth control

Some women get pregnant again only a few months after birth. Most do not want to be pregnant so soon. This can be very hard on their health and that of their baby.

Family planning means deciding when you and your partner want another baby. It means using birth control (contraception or protection) to make sure you do not get pregnant before you are ready. Ask yourselves how many children you want. When do you want another baby?

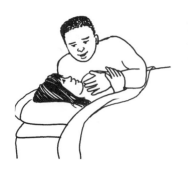

It is best to have your babies at least 18 months to 2 years apart. This gives your body time to get strong again after birth. It also helps your babies be healthier. This would mean waiting to get pregnant until your baby is at least 9 to 15 months of age.

Facts about family planning

- A woman can get pregnant before her menstrual periods start again.

- **Breastfeeding is not an effective form of birth control** for more than the first few months. It can work for a few months if you breastfeed exclusively and give no other food or water to your baby. For long-term protection from pregnancy, you need to use a different contraceptive method.

- **Withdrawal** of the man's penis before orgasm is not effective.

- **The rhythm method** can only be used after your periods are completely regular again.

- **If you start having sex before you see your doctor,** use condoms and spermicide* (foam or jelly) together, or a spermicidal sponge. They cost very little and are available at drug stores without a prescription. These are not as effective as other methods for long-term use.

  *Spermicide: Medication that kills the male sperm.

- **The condom** is the only kind of birth control that also can prevent sexually-transmitted diseases. There are condoms for women as well as for men.

- **Many kinds of birth control are very safe,** easy to use, and effective. Talk with your doctor or nurse midwife about the choices you have, such as the pill, injection, patch, IUD, and diaphragm. All have different benefits.

Emergency contraception

If you have had sex without protection (or if a condom breaks), there is an emergency pill. It can keep you from getting pregnant if taken within two to three days of having unprotected sex. Call your health care provider and ask about emergency contraception. It is only for emergencies, not to be used instead of a regular birth control method.

Feeling unhappy or depressed?

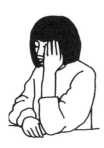

The days after delivery can be very emotional. There are so many new things to learn and so much responsibility. What others think is a happy time can be very difficult.

Many women feel upset or sad after they give birth. They may cry easily, get angry over little things, or have trouble eating and sleeping. This is normal and usually goes away in about two weeks.

These feelings come partly from the changes in your hormones after birth. Also, you probably are not getting enough sleep. You may find being a parent a lot more work and less fun than you had dreamed. You may feel very alone and miss your friends at work. It is okay to cry about these things.

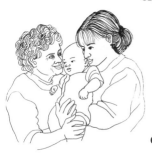

Being a new parent can be hard, even though you are getting to know and love your baby. Tell your partner, relatives, and friends when you are feeling low. Sometimes, simply telling someone about your feelings can make you feel better.

If your unhappiness lasts more than two weeks, check for these signs of depression:

- Feeling very sad, guilty, or hopeless
- Feeling like you are not able to care for your baby
- Worrying about things that you can't do anything about
- Sleeping all day or not sleeping much at all
- Being unable to eat
- Feeling like you cannot concentrate on what you are doing
- Feeling that you might hurt yourself or your baby

If you feel even one or two of the feelings above, you should get help. Depression can easily happen. It does not mean you are a poor parent, so do not be shy about asking for help.

Talk with your partner or a friend. Call your doctor or nurse or a mental health counselor. Deal with depression as soon as possible. Your baby needs your love and attention. You deserve to enjoy your baby and this special time in your life.

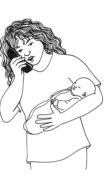

No one is a perfect parent!

Are you or your partner worried about doing things wrong? You do not have to know all the answers. You will learn as you go along.

You can get advice from friends, relatives, neighbors, your health clinic, and many organizations. There are parent groups, breast-feeding consultants, and playgroups to turn to. Books, videos, and the Internet have a wealth of good information.

Remember, every community has resources to help parents raise happy, healthy children. **You do not have to do it alone!**

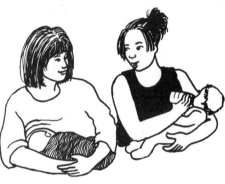

Affirmations to remember

I am learning more every day about being good to myself.

I'm not the first person who has gone through this special—and sometimes difficult—time.

I have friends I can call on when I need support or someone to talk with.

I know I can find people in the community to help if I need it.

I am learning more every day about how to be a parent.

I am being the best parent I can be, knowing what I know now.

I see how my baby learns and grows from week to week.

My baby gives me the chance to become a new person.

Nobody is perfect. My child will forgive the small mistakes I make.

Nothing ever stays the same. Each day brings a new chance to grow.

I am a good mother.

Chapter 17

Resources to Help You

When you need to know more

There's more to know about pregnancy, birth, and infant care than could be put into one book. This chapter gives you the tools to learn more.

If you hear or read advice that seems completely different from what you have read here or heard from your health care provider, be sure to check it. Ask your health care provider about what you learn. Use your common sense before making big changes in what you do.

I'm glad you have completed your pregnancy and wish you success as a parent. I hope this book has helped you. If you would like to buy a copy for a friend or relative, please call Bull Publishing at 1-800-676-2855.

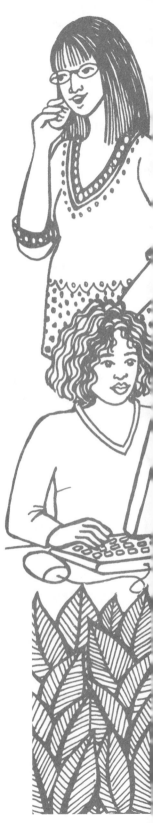

This chapter includes:

Organizations, page 224

- Help in your community
- National groups

Books, page 228

- Pregnancy
- Baby care

Glossary: meanings of words, page 229

Index: finding information in this book, page 236

Getting Help

You may already know about some of the organizations listed here. They all have useful services for pregnant women and new parents. They can help you find other resources. Many can be found on the Internet (see National Resources list).

Some of the best help will come from organizations or agencies in your own city or town. Most national organizations have local chapters. Their phone numbers and addresses can be found in your Yellow Pages or White Pages. Look under "Health," "Education," or "Government" listings.

You also can find local links on national organization Web sites. Your health care provider, county health department, or hospital social worker will also be able to help.

Community resources:

Breastfeeding (Lactation) consultants, La Leche League

Certified nurse-midwives and doulas

Childbirth education classes, ICEA, Lamaze

Church, synagogue, or other place of worship: Parent support programs.

Community health centers: Prenatal and well-baby care.

Community colleges: Parent education.

Community information lines: Referral to local services, available in many cities and counties.

County Health Department: Prenatal care, well-baby care, parent education, home visits.

Crisis hotline: Telephone help and information service for people who are very upset, sad, or angry, including abused women.

Family planning: Planned Parenthood clinics.

Hospitals: Childbirth preparation classes, parenting and infant first aid classes.

Mental health center: Counseling and support groups for people with problems.

Parent support groups: Groups set up by different organizations where parents support and help one another. Includes groups of new parents and groups of parents of children with specific disabilities.

Public library: Books, pamphlets, tapes, and notices of educational programs on prenatal and family health.

Safe Kids Coalition: car seat and other child safety information and programs.

School nurse: Health care professional who is able to help students deal with health challenges.

WIC: Women, Infant, and Children Food and Nutrition Program.

Your health plan: Your health insurance company or HMO, which may include a health information service.

National resources:

There is an amazing amount of excellent information on the Internet. There is also questionable information. If you do not have a computer and need to contact one of those organizations, you can use a computer at a local library.

Some Web pages will have useful links to other helpful sites. Some also have Spanish-language pages.

Internet addresses may change unexpectedly. If you cannot locate the service you want from the address given here, please search using key words like the name of the organization or a specific topic such as "breastfeeding information."

Be careful when using the Internet. Check out the sponsors of the sites you find and the sources of information. Look first at sites from major medical or government organizations. Some other sites are by smaller non-profit groups, but others mainly sell products. Some give only one side of a health issue, one that may be not medically accurate. If you find information that is very different from what is in this book, be sure to ask about it at your next checkup.

Alcohol, drug, tobacco abuse:

National Drug and Substance Abuse Treatment Hotline 1-800-662-HELP (1-800-662-4357)

Tobacco Information and Prevention Source: guide to quitting smoking; http://www.cdc.gov/tobacco /quit/canquit.htm

National Clearinghouse for Alcohol and Drug Information: 1-800-729-6686

Breastfeeding

La Leche League: Information and help with breastfeeding, or to find a local group or leader; http://www.lalecheleague.org, 1-800-LALECHE (1-800-525-3243)

National Women's Health Information Center: http:www.4woman.gov /Breastfeeding/

American Academy of Pediatrics: http://www.aap.org/healthtopics /breastfeeding.cfm

Child abuse:

National Clearinghouse on Child Abuse and Neglect Information, http://nccanch.acf.hhs.gov/

National Child Abuse Hotline: 1-800-4-A-CHILD (1-800-422-4453)

Childbirth education:

International Childbirth Education Association (ICEA): Classes in childbirth preparation and parenting. Find childbirth teachers, http://www.icea.org

Lamaze International: Classes in Lamaze method of childbirth; preparation and parenting; Find local teachers: http://www.lamaze.org; 1-800-368-4404

Depression (postpartum depression):

National Women's Health Information Center: http://www.4woman.gov/faq/postpartum.htm

Domestic violence:

Women'sLaw.org: state-by-state legal information and resources for abused women, http://www.womenslaw.org/

National Domestic Violence Hotline, 1-800-799-SAFE (1-800-799-7233), also Spanish service; http://www.ndvh.org/

State hotlines or local crisis center hotlines.

Doulas of North America:

Trained birth helpers: http://www.dona.org; 1-888-788-DONA (1-888-788-3662)

Family planning:

Planned Parenthood Federation of America: birth control, family planning, women's health; (phone number connects a caller with the nearest clinic), 1-800-230-PLAN (1-800-230-7526), http://www.plannedparenthood.org/womenshealth/

Infant health and development:

American Academy of Pediatrics: select health topics or search, http://www.aap.org/topics.html and http://www.aap.org/parents.html

American Academy of Family Physicians: http://www.familydoctor.org

Kids Health (Nemours Foundation): http:www.kidshealth.org

Zero to Three: child development, http://zerotothree.org/ztt_parents.html

Tufts University Child and Family WebGuide: http://www.cfw.tufts.edu

Injury prevention, general child-related:

Safe Kids U.S.A.: http://www.safekids.org, 202-662-0600

Nutrition, food safety:

Healthy eating, New food pyramid: includes how to find out what to eat based on age and activity level, http://www.mypyramid.gov/

WIC (Special Supplemental Nutrition Program for Women, Infants, and Children), http://www.fns.usda.gov/wic/ (click on "How to Apply" to find state contacts and toll-free numbers)

Mercury in fish: http://www.epa.gov/waterscience/fish/index.html

Poisoning help, advice:

(NOTE: If the victim has collapsed or is not breathing, call 9-1-1 immediately)

National hotline, 1-800-222-1222

American Association of Poison Control Centers, http://www.aapcc.org /children.htm

Pregnancy and Childbirth

American College of Nurse-Midwives: http://www.midwife.org/focus/

March of Dimes: Prenatal education and information on birth defects; http://www.marchofdimes.com/

Maternity Center Association: clear discussions of current issues, like non-emergency cesarean delivery, based on current research; (212) 777-5000, http://www.maternitywise.org,

National Women's Health Information Center: pregnancy, breastfeeding, etc.; 800-994-WOMAN (9662); http://www.4woman.gov/ pregnancy/

Safety in the car:

SafetyBeltSafe U.S.A., Helpline:1-800-745-SAFE (1-800-745-7233); http://www.carseat.org

National Highway Traffic Safety Administration, car seat information, recalls, Auto Safety Hotline, 1-800-424-9393; http://www.nhtsa.dot.gov/cps/

Car Seat Checkup (inspection) site locator: http://www.seatcheck.org/; 1-866-SEAT-CHECK (1-866-732-8243)

Car seat safety links: http://www.cpsafety.com

Safety at home:

Consumer Product Safety Commission: Safety information and recalls of children's furniture and toys, http://www.cpsc.gov, 1-800-638-2772

Home Safety Council: http://www.homesafetycouncil.org

Sudden Infant Death Syndrome:

- SIDS: Back to Sleep Campaign; http://www.nichd.nih.gov/sids /sids.htm

- SIDS alliance: http://www.sidsalliance.org

Teen parents:

http://www.cfw.tufts.edu (go to Family/Parenting)

http://www.teenparents.org/

http://www.teenageparent.org/

Twins, Multiples:

Mothers of Twins Clubs: Support for families with twins and multiple births; http://www.nomotc.org/

WIC Food and Nutrition Program:

See Nutrition listing above

Women's Health:

Nat'l Women's Health Information Center: http://www.4woman.gov/

Choices for further reading

This book has given you the basics every woman needs to know during pregnancy and the first months after birth. There are many books that have more details. Here are a few books that I think you would find useful. Find them in your library or local bookstores or Planned Parenthood bookstores.

Some books about general baby care, behavior, or development are classic. They do not really go out of date. However, when choosing a book for medical care information, make sure it was published in the last few years. (Check the date on the back of the title page.) If you find advice that confuses you, be sure to ask your doctor or nurse midwife about it.

Look for books from medical organizations and from well-known authors, such as T. Berry Brazelton, MD; William Sears, MD; Penelope Leach; Penny Simkin; and Sheila Kitzinger. Open a book and read a few pages before buying it. Compare something specific, like breastfeeding, in several books. Some will be easier or more fun to read than others.

Prenatal Care

A Child is Born, Lennart Nilsson, 2003, a classic book of photographs of conception, pregnancy, birth

Complete Book of Pregnancy and Childbirth, Sheila Kitzinger, 2004, **Girlfriends' Guide to Pregnancy,** Vicki Iovine, 1995, humorous and practical

K.I.S.S. Guide to Pregnancy, Felicia Molnar, 2001, easy to read, clear summaries, excellent photos

Nine Months and a Day, Annette Lieberman and Linda Hold, MD, 2000

Pregnancy, Childbirth and the Newborn, Penny Simkin, PT, Janet Whalley, RN, BSN, and Ann Keppler, RN, MN, 2001

When You're Expecting Twins, Triplets, or Quads, Dr. Barbara Luke & Tamara Eberlein, 2004

Especially For Teens

Your Pregnancy & Newborn Journey: A Guide for Pregnant Teens

Nurturing Your Newborn: Young Parents' Guide to Baby's First Month

Teen Dads: Rights, Responsibilities & Joys

Your Baby's First Year, A Guide for Teenage Parents,

These book are from Morning Glory Press, by Jeanne Lindsay and Jean Brunelli, PHN, http://www.morningglorypress.com

Baby Care

Best Start, Your Baby's First Year, Deborah Stewart and Linda Ungerleider, 2001, Bull Publishing

Heading Home with your Newborn, Laura A. Jana, MD, and Jennifer Shu, MD, 2005, American Academy of Pediatrics

Caring for Your Baby and Young Child, Steven P. Shelov and Robert E. Hanneman, Editors, 4th Edition, 2004, American Academy of Pediatrics

Breastfeeding, Pure & Simple, Gwen Gotsch, 1994, La Leche League International

Girlfriends' Guide to Surviving the First Year of Motherhood, Vicki Iovine, 1997, humorous and practical

K.I.S.S. Guide to Baby & Child Care, Joanna Moorhead, 2002, easy to read, clear summaries, excellent photos

Premature Baby Book, William Sears, MD and others, 2004,

The Womanly Art of Breastfeeding, La Leche League, 2004, a classic book

Touchpoints: Your Child's Emotional and Behavioral Development, T. Berry Brazelton, MD, 1992, a classic book, as are others by Dr. Brazelton

Year After Childbirth: Surviving and Enjoying the First Year of Motherhood, Sheila Kitzinger, 1994

A Glossary of Words to Know

Abdomen – The part of your body below your ribs and above your legs. Contains your stomach, uterus, and other organs.

Abortion – Ending of a pregnancy, which may be natural (miscarriage) or done by a doctor (induced).

AIDS – Short word for Acquired Immunodeficiency Syndrome, a fatal disease passed from person to person most often by having sex or sharing needles. May be passed to an unborn baby.

Air Bag – A safety device for front seat car passengers that is hidden in the dashboard and opens if a crash occurs.

Amniocentesis – A test of the fluid inside the bag of waters, showing certain things about your unborn baby's health.

Amniotic fluid – Liquid in the amniotic sac.

Amniotic sac – The "bag of waters" inside the uterus, in which the baby grows.

Anesthesia – Various drugs used to reduce or eliminate pain.

Antibodies – Cells made in a person's body to fight disease. A baby's first antibodies come from mother's colostrum and milk.

Aspirin – A drug you can buy without a doctor's prescription that lessens pain and lowers fever.

Areola – The dark area around the nipple.

Bag of waters – The amniotic sac in which your baby grows inside the uterus.

Birth canal – Your vagina, the opening through which your baby will be born.

Birth control – Ways to keep from becoming pregnant when you have sex. Examples: condom, diaphragm, pills, IUD.

Birth defect – Baby's health problem that happens before birth or during birth. May have lasting effects.

Blood pressure – The force of blood pumped by the heart through a person's blood vessels. High blood pressure means the heart is pumping extra hard.

Bloody show – A small amount of mucus and blood (the "mucus plug") that comes from your cervix before labor begins.

Braxton-Hicks contractions – Tightening and relaxing of the muscle of your uterus during the last few months of pregnancy.

Breech birth – Birth of a baby with buttocks first.

Calcium – A mineral in foods needed to make bones and teeth grow strong.

Calories – Energy in foods. Some kinds of foods have more calories than others.

Car seat – A seat specially designed and tested for use to protect infants or children from injury in a vehicle crash.

Certified Nurse-midwife – A nurse who delivers babies, who has been specially trained as a midwife and passed a national test.

Cervix – The neck (opening) of the uterus (womb). Your baby is pushed out through the cervix into the vagina during delivery.

Cesarean section – Delivery of a baby by making a cut through the woman's belly into the uterus.

Child safety seat (child restraint) – Other words for "car seat".

Circumcision – Surgery to take off the loose skin around the top of a baby boy's penis.

Colostrum – The thin, yellowish liquid that comes out of a woman's nipples during late pregnancy and the first few days after birth.

Conception – The beginning of a baby's growth, when the mother's egg unites with the father's sperm.

Condom – A rubber or latex tube with a closed end that is put on a man's penis during sex to prevent pregnancy and diseases that can be passed during sex.

Constipation – When bowel movements are very hard and do not come regularly.

Contraception – See Birth control.

Contractions – The tightening and relaxing of the muscle of your uterus.

Development – The ways in which the baby's mind learns and the body grows and changes.

Diarrhea – Bowel movements that are very soft and watery and come more often than usual.

Digestion – The changing of your food in your mouth, stomach, and intestines for use by your body.

Dilation – The stretching open of the cervix during the first stage of labor.

Discharge – Liquid that comes out of your body, like blood or mucus from your vagina.

Doula – A person trained to help parents during and after delivery.

Drop – The sinking of the unborn baby down into the pelvis before birth begins.

Drugs – Many kinds of things that affect your body or feelings, such as medicines, or substances like alcohol, tobacco, or illegal (street) drugs.

Effacement – The thinning of the cervix during the first stage of labor.

Embryo – Word used for a tiny unborn baby during the first eight weeks of its growth.

Engagement – The sinking (dropping) of the uterus down into the pelvis before birth.

Engorgement – Hard and painful breasts when they are starting to produce milk.

Episiotomy – A cut made in the skin around the vagina to widen the opening and help the baby to be born.

Family physician or practitioner – A doctor who takes care of the health of people of all ages.

Family planning – Using a birth control method to control the number of children in the family, and getting pregnant when a person or couple chooses.

Fetal monitoring – A machine that tells how the unborn baby's heart is beating, used to check the baby's health inside the uterus.

Fetus – Word used for the unborn baby, from 8 weeks to birth at about 40 weeks.

Fiber – A substance in foods that helps bowel movements be soft and come regularly.

Fontanelles – Soft spots in the skull of a newborn baby. They close gradually over many months.

Formula – Special milk for bottle-feeding. Made to be much like breast milk.

Genetic counseling – Help for people with health problems that may be passed down to their children.

Genetic defects – Health problems that are passed down from parent to child to grandchild through genetic matter in the cells.

Genitals – A boy's penis and girl's vulva.

Gestational Diabetes – A type of diabetes that happens during pregnancy and can cause problems for mother and baby if not found and controlled.

Group B Streptococcus (GBS) – A type of bacteria ("Strep") that can live in the vagina and can seriously harm a newborn baby.

Health care provider – A person trained to take care of people's health and illness (nurses, doctors, nurse-midwives).

Heartburn – A burning feeling in your chest caused by acid from your stomach going up into the tube from your mouth.

Hemorrhoids – Veins at your anus (opening where bowel movements come out) that get swollen and feel itchy or painful.

Hormones – Substances made by organs in the body that control how it works and feels.

Immune system – The body system that fights disease by making antibodies.

Immunization (vaccination, shot) – Injection (or other application) of a vaccine that helps the body make antibodies to fight against a disease.

Infection – A sore or illness caused by germs that harm your body.

Iron – A mineral in foods that helps your blood carry oxygen to your baby's body.

Isopropyl alcohol – The kind of alcohol used to kill germs (not safe to drink).

Kangaroo care – Cuddling a baby against the parent's bare chest so they are skin-to-skin. Especially comforting for premies.

Labor – The work your uterus does to open the cervix and push the baby down into the birth canal.

Lactation Specialist – A nurse with special knowledge about breastfeeding (lactation).

LATCH system – Lower Anchors and Tethers for Children; a new method of installing a car seat in a vehicle using special connectors on the car seat and anchors in the vehicle.

Lanugo – Soft, short hair growing on the body of a fetus and newborn baby.

Medication – Drugs (medicines) that a doctor prescribes for you or that you can buy at a drug store.

Menstrual period – The bloody lining of the uterus that flows from a woman's vagina every month.

Midwife – A person who helps women have their babies. Not a doctor.

Miscarriage (spontaneous abortion) – Delivery of a dead embryo or fetus earlier than about 20 weeks, too early to survive.

Morning sickness – Name for feeling of nausea, often with vomiting, in the first few months of pregnancy.

Mucus plug – The thick blob of material that fills the cervix during pregnancy.

Multiple pregnancy – Twins, triplets, or more babies born at the same time.

Neonatal Intensive Care Unit (NICU) – The hospital nursery for preterm infants or those with serious medical problems.

Non-aspirin pain reliever – Acetaminophen, a drug better than aspirin for children with pain or fever; "Tylenol" is one common brand.

Nurse-midwife – A nurse with special training to deliver babies.

Nurse practitioner – A nurse with special training to do some aspects of health care, working with a doctor.

Nursing – Another word for breastfeeding.

Nutrients – Things in foods that keep you healthy.

Obstetrician-Gynecologist – A doctor who takes care of women's health. An obstetrician specializes in prenatal care and delivery of babies. A gynecologist specializes in the health of women's uterus and sex organs.

Pelvis – Your hip bones inside which your uterus sits. Your vagina (birth canal) goes through a wide opening in these bones.

Pediatrician – A doctor who takes care of children's health.

Pelvic exam – A way for your doctor or nurse midwife to check your vagina and uterus by pressing on your belly and reaching up inside your vagina, and by looking inside.

Perineum – The skin and muscles around the opening of the vagina.

Period – A short word for menstrual period.

Placenta – The organ that connects the mother's body with her fetus, moving food and oxygen from the mother's blood to the unborn baby's blood.

Pregnancy – The nine months when a woman has a baby growing inside her uterus.

Pregnancy-induced hypertension (PIH) – High blood pressure during pregnancy. May lead to preeclampsia if not treated.

Premie – Short term for a preterm infant.

Preterm (premature) – A baby born early, before 37 weeks of gestation (growth in the uterus).

Prenatal – Nine-month period when a baby is growing in the mother.

Prescription – An order for medicine from your doctor.

Protein – Substances in food that make your body grow well and work properly.

Reflexes – Movements of the body that happen automatically.

Reflux – Acid from the stomach that backs up into the esophagus (tube from the mouth to the stomach).

Sexually-transmitted disease (STD) – A disease passed from one person to another when they have sex.

Spinal cord – The main nerve in the body that goes up the middle of the spine or backbone. It connects the brain to the rest of the body.

Stool – Another term for a bowel movement.

Sudden infant death syndrome (SIDS or crib death) – Mysterious death of a sleeping baby when all other causes have been ruled out.

Support system – The people in your life or community who help you in times of need.

Swaddling – Wrapping a newborn baby snugly in a thin blanket for comfort.

Symptoms – Changes in your body or how you feel (like pain, itching, or bleeding). These help a doctor or nurse midwife know what health problem you have.

Trimester – A three-month period. The nine months of pregnancy are divided into three trimesters.

Ultrasound – Special tool used to see inside your body to find out how your unborn baby is growing. It uses a rounded wand that is moved around on your belly. The images show on a screen.

Umbilical cord – The long tube that attaches the placenta to the unborn baby's body at the navel or belly button. It carries food and oxygen from the mother's body and wastes from the baby's body.

Uterus – The womb, the organ in which an unborn baby grows.

Vaccine – Substance given to immunize against disease.

Vagina – The opening in a woman's body where menstrual flow comes out and a man puts his penis during sex. Also, the birth canal through which a baby is born.

Vaginal birth – The natural type of birth, in which the baby passes through the cervix and vagina.

Varicose veins – Blue, swollen veins that itch or ache, that often occur in the legs during pregnancy.

VBAC – A short word for Vaginal Birth After a Cesarean.

Vernix – Grayish-white, cheese-like substance covering the skin of a newborn baby.

Vomiting – Throwing up stomach contents.

Vulva – The female genitals around the opening of the vagina.

Well-baby, Well-child checkup – Regular health visits for babies and children who are not ill. Checkups cover health, development, immunizations, and screening tests.

WIC (Women, Infants, and Children) Program – A federal nutrition program that provides food and educational support for eligible pregnant women and children up to age 5.

Index

Abortion, spontaneous 89
Abuse, 29-30
    alcohol/drug, 225
    child, 225
Affirmations, 222
Air bag, 194-195
Alcohol, 2, 4, 5, 42–44, 79, 191, 217
Amniocentesis, 90
Amniotic
    fluid, 74
    sac, 74
Anencephaly, 6
Antibiotics, 210–222

Baby-proofing, 197–198
Backache, 89, 95, 101
Bathing, 158–160
Beans, 33
Behavior, infant, 180–181
Birth, 127–148
    center, 49
    control, 4, 218–219
        and breastfeeding, 219
        emergency, 219
    defects, 90
    and newborn care, 55–70
    partner, 56–57, 60
        tips for, 133–134
    plan, 119–120
    preparing for, 128–129
    preterm (premature), 145
    recovery from, 144
    stages of, 135–144
    vaginal, 142, 143
Bleeding, 88, 89, 101, 214, 215
Blood pressure, high, 3, 111
Bottle feeding, 174–176
Bradley childbirth method, 57
Brain damage, 26
Braxton Hicks contractions, 116
Breads, 33
Breastfeeding, 61–64, 102, 147, 151, 154,
    166–174, 191, 199, 224, 225
    and birth control, 219
    pumping, 172
    quitting, 217
    twins, 171
Breasts, 167
    caring for, 172–172, 216
    painful, 97, 215

Breathing problems, 155
Breech, 117
Brothers and sisters, 179
Burns, preventing, 197
Burping, 165

Caffeine, 38
Calcium, 33, 36–37
Carbohydrates, 32
Car
    bed, 196
    crashes, 189
    safety seat, 25, 65, 68, 69–70, 154,
        184, 185, 193–196
        installing, 193–194
Cesarean section, 51, 57, 58, 59, 88, 117,
    132–133, 146
    recovery from, 216
    risks of, 59
Checkups, 51–52, 75–77, 83, 84, 92, 93,
    98, 99, 105, 110, 111, 113, 114, 116,
    123, 124, 125, 218
    baby's, 201–202
Chicken pox, 205
Childbirth education, 57, 128, 225–226
Chlamydia, 3
Circumcision, 113
Clothes, 65
Colic, 188
Colostrum, 116, 168
Condom, 26, 219
Constipation, 82, 101, 215
Contraception, 4, 218–219
Contractions, 101, 130, 131
    Braxton Hicks, 100, 116
    keeping track of, 138
Coughing, 207
Cramps, 88, 89, 101
Crib/cradle, 65–66, 68–69
Crying, 187
C-section. See Cesarean section
Cystic fibrosis, 3

Dairy, 33
Delivery
    cesarean, 132–133
    vaginal (VBAC), 59–60, 133
    sudden/unexpected, 131–132
Dental care, 22, 79, 160
Depression, 179, 220–221, 226

Development, 182
   delays in, 185
   milestones in, 186
Diabetes, 3, 106
Diapers, 65, 153
   rash, preventing, 157
Diarrhea, 155, 156, 207, 209
Dilation, 117
Diphtheria, 204
Discharge, 214, 215
Dizziness, 88
Domestic violence, 30, 226
Doula, 60, 226
Driving, 23–25
   and drinking, 44
Drugs, illegal, 3, 42, 46, 191, 217–218
DTaP, 204

Eating
   for two, 85–86
   healthy, 32–37
Effacement, 117
Eggs, 33
Embryo, 74
Emergency
   room, 211
   signs of, 88
Epidural block, 141–142
Episiotomy, 51, 144, 214, 215
   avoiding, 115, 118
Exercise, 22–23, 32, 92, 95–96, 98, 101,
     104, 110, 112, 118, 123, 188, 217

Falling, protection from, 196
Family, 180
   physician, 49
   planning, 218, 226
Father, 14–15, 102–103, 178–179
Feeding, 151, 163–176
   bottle, 174–176
   breast-, 61–64, 102, 147, 151, 154,
     166–174, 191, 199, 224, 225
   formula, 175–176
   hunger signs, 164
Fetal Alcohol Syndrome, 42, 43
Fetus, 74
Fever, 88, 153, 207, 208, 209–210, 215
Fiber, 32
Fish, 33, 39–40
Flat spot on head, 184–185, 192
Flu, 204, 205
Folic acid, 4, 5–6, 36
Fontanel, 150
Food
   healthy, 33–34
   safety, 40–41
Formula feeding, 64, 175–176
Fruit, 33

Gates, 69
Glossary, 229–235
Gonorrhea, 3
Growth, baby's, 20
Gums, caring for, 160

Habits
   breaking bad, 79
   healthy, 86–87
Hand washing, 153, 154, 200–201
Headaches, 88
Health
   baby's, 199–212
   care provider
     choosing, 49–51
     talking with, 52–53
   caring for your, 17–30, 92–93,
     98, 104, 110, 112, 123,
     213–222
Heartburn, 94
Hemophilia, 3
Hepatitis
   A, 204, 205
   B, 201, 204, 205
Herpes, 3
Hib, 204
High blood pressure, 3, 111
HIV/AIDS, 3
Holding baby, 169, 185
Hormones, 80
Hospitals, 48
Hot tub/sauna, 27
Household hazards, 26–27
Hunger, signs of, 181

Illness, 206–211
Immunizations, 200, 202–206
   recommended, 204
   side effects, 206
Infant health, 226
Influenza, 204, 205
Injury prevention, 226
Insurance, 47, 48, 54
Iron, 37

Jaundice, 209
Job and pregnancy, 27–28

Kangaroo care, 153, 161
Kegel squeeze, 95, 214
Kicking, 114–115
Knowing your baby, 177–188

Labor, 57, 135, 136–142
   early, 136
   false, 131
   inducing, 132
   preparing for, 129–130

preterm, 100, 101, 109
   signs of, 101, 121, 130
Lactation consultant, 151, 166, 171
Lactose intolerance, 36
La Leche League, 167, 171
LaMaze childbirth method, 57
Lanugo, 150
Lead, 26–27
Legs, swollen, 94, 215
Lifting objects, 96
Listeriosis, 41

Mastitis, 173
Maternity leave, 61
Measles, 203, 204, 205
Medical care, 47–54
Medicine, 42
   giving, 210–211
Mercury, 39–40
Milia, 150
Milk, hind (breast), 168–169
Minerals, 32
Miscarriage, 3, 12, 26, 41, 44, 46, 89
MMR, 204, 205
Mood swings, 80–81
Morning sickness, 78–79
Mucus plug, 101, 130
Multiples, 88, 180, 228
Mumps, 204, 205

National Domestic Violence Hotline, 30
Nausea, 78–79
Newborn care
   activity, 150
   appearance, 150
   bathing, 158–160
   birth, 55–70
   dressing, 160
   feeding, 151, 163–176
   holding, 152, 155–156
   keeping clean, 156–160
   safety, 154
NICU (newborn intensive care unit), 161,
   162
Nipple shapes, 102
Nurse-midwife, 49
Nursing. See Breastfeeding
Nuts, 33

Obstetrician-gynecologist (OB-Gyn), 49
Oils, 33
Over 35 years old, 13

Pacifiers, 171, 191
Pain, 58, 59, 140
   medications, 141–142
Partner, information for, 14–15
PCV, 204, 205

Pediatrician, choosing, 53–54, 113
Pelvic
   exam, 52
   tilt, 95
Penis, cleaning a circumcised, 157
Perineum, massaging the, 115,
   118
Period, menstrual, 6, 7
Personality, 181
Pertussis, 204
PIH, 111
Placenta, 74, 135, 144
Planned Parenthood, 7
Playing with baby, 183–184
Playpen, 69
Polio, 204, 205
Poisoning, 227
Poultry, 33
Preeclampsia, 111
Pregnancy
   effects on your body, 92, 98, 103,
      108–109, 112, 122
   growth during, 73, 92, 98, 104, 109,
      112, 122
   and job, 27–28
   length of, 72
   preparing for, 1–8
   signs of, 6, 10
   test, 7
Premature (preterm) birth, 5, 145, 184,
   196
Prenatal
   care, 12, 18–19
   checkups, 51–52, 75–77, 83, 84, 92,
      93, 98, 99, 105, 110, 111, 113,
      114, 116, 123, 124, 125
   vitamins, 37–38
Problems, preventing, 2–6
Protein, 32
Pumping, 172, 173–174

Reflux, 187
Relaxation, 28–29
Resources, 223–235
Rh negative, 106
Rotavirus, 209
RSV, 209

Safety, 189–198
   car, 227
   food, 226
   home, 227
Sauna, 27
Seat belts, 23–25
Seizures, 3
Serving sizes, 34–35
Sex, 97, 103
   safe, 25

Sexually transmitted disease (STD), 3, 25–26, 97, 219
Shaking, 185, 188
Sharing a bed with baby, 191–192
Shots, 200, 202–206
    recommended, 204
    side effects, 206
Sickle cell disease, 3
Sickness, signs of, 206–211
Single woman (mom), 13
Sleep
    baby's, 186–187
    problems, 215
    signs a baby needs, 181
Smoke detectors, 197
Smoking, 2, 5, 79, 191, 200, 218
Snacks, healthy, 94
Social worker, 162
Spermicide, 26
Spina bifida, 6
Stitches, 214
Strep infection, 115
Stress, 28–29
Sudden Infant Death Syndrome (SIDS), 154, 189, 218, 227
    preventing, 190–192
Sunburn, 160–161, 197
Sun protection, 160–161
Supplements, 39
Supplies
    helpful, 66–67
    second-hand, 68–69
Swaddling, 152
Swelling, 88
Swollen legs, 94, 215
Syphillis, 3

Talking to baby, 182–183
Tay-Sachs disease, 3
Teen parent, 13, 227
Teeth, brushing, 22, 79, 160

Tetanus, 204
Tiredness, 78
Tobacco, 4, 42, 44–46. *See also* Smoking
Toothpaste, 160
Toxemia, 111
Trimester
    first, 71–90
    second, 91–106
    third, 107–126
Triplets, 180, 228
Tummy time, 184
Twins, 88, 180, 228

Ultrasound, 11
Umbilical cord, 74
    stump, caring for, 158
Upset stomach, 78–79
Uterus, 74

Vaccines. *See* Immunizations
Vaginal birth after delivery (VBAC), 59–60
Varicella, 204, 205
Vegetables, 33
Vegetarian, 36
Vitamins, 32
    prenatal, 37–38
Vomiting, 155, 156, 207, 209

Walking, 22–23
Warning signs, health, 215
Water, 32, 34
    breaks, 130, 131
Weight
    body, 4
    gain, 85–86
    low birth, 145–146
Whooping cough, 203
WIC, 40, 228

X-ray, 27